PHARMA MARKETING MANAGEMENT

PHARMA MARKETING MANAGEMENT

BY

ELSEA LEWIS
SIENNA PHILLIPS

KNOWLEDGE
BAKERS

KNOWLEDGE BAKERS

ISBN: 978-81-9759-573-8 (HB)

Published by : **Knowledge Bakers**
Pune, India
Email: info@knowledgebakers.com

PREFACE

Pharmaceutical marketing management plays a pivotal role in navigating the complex landscape of the healthcare industry, where the convergence of medical science, regulatory frameworks, and market dynamics shapes the success of pharmaceutical products and services. As the pharmaceutical sector continues to evolve amidst technological advancements, shifting consumer behaviors, and regulatory changes, effective marketing strategies and management practices are essential for pharmaceutical companies to succeed in delivering value to patients, healthcare providers, and stakeholders. As we embark on this exploration of pharma marketing management, we delve into a realm where healthcare innovation, commercial strategy, and ethical considerations intersect, uncovering the principles, methodologies, and challenges that define marketing in the pharmaceutical industry.

This book, titled "Pharma Marketing Management," is crafted to provide a comprehensive overview of the principles, strategies, and best practices in pharmaceutical marketing management. Through collaboration with leading experts, practitioners, and thought leaders in the pharmaceutical and healthcare sectors, we aim to offer readers a multidimensional and insightful journey through the intricacies of marketing pharmaceutical products and services.

As editors of this volume, we have curated a collection of chapters that cover a wide range of topics in pharma marketing management, including market analysis, product positioning, branding, promotion, pricing, distribution, regulatory compliance, digital marketing, and market access strategies. Each chapter is designed to provide theoretical insights, practical strategies, case studies, and examples to empower readers to navigate the complexities of marketing pharmaceutical products in diverse markets and therapeutic areas.

Furthermore, this book seeks to highlight the evolving landscape of pharmaceutical marketing and its implications for healthcare stakeholders. By exploring the impact of digital technologies, patient-centric approaches, and value-based healthcare models on pharmaceutical marketing practices, we aim to inspire readers to adopt innovative strategies and ethical principles that drive value creation, patient engagement, and healthcare outcomes.

As we embark on this enlightening journey through the world of pharma marketing management, we extend our gratitude to the contributors whose expertise and dedication have enriched this book. We hope that "Pharma Marketing Management" serves as a valuable resource for professionals, executives, researchers, and students in the pharmaceutical and healthcare industries, empowering them to navigate the challenges and opportunities of pharmaceutical marketing with integrity, innovation, and strategic insight.

Elsea Lewis
Sienna Phillips

CONTENTS

1

Pharma Marketing: Introduction

Pharmaceutical company spending on marketing generally exceeds that of its research budget. In Canada, \$1.7 billion was spent in 2004 to market drugs to physicians; in the United States, \$21 billion was spent in 2002. In 2005, money spent on pharmaceutical marketing in the United States was estimated at \$29.9 billion with one estimate as high as \$57 billion. When the U.S. numbers are broken down, 56% was free samples, 25% was pharmaceutical sales representative "detailing" (promoting drugs directly to) physicians, 12.5% was direct to user advertising, 4% on detailing to hospitals, and 2% on journal ads. There is some evidence that marketing practices can negatively affect both patients and the health care profession.

1. Marketing's Role in Pharma

Textbooks will define marketing's role as the process that starts with identifying and understanding the needs and wants of the customer (demand) and then fulfilling those needs and wants (supply). Broadly speaking, pharmaceutical marketing involves all of the promotional activities carried out by an organisation to make pharmaceutical products and care a reality, and available to customers (patients and other decision makers) from the manufacturer.

Within the pharmaceutical manufacturing sectors - which Orientation Marketing predominantly operate within - marketing will refer to the promotional activities carried out between the organisations that produce the various products and services that complete the supply chain. The patient sits at the top of the chain, who can access pharmaceutical care from HCPs provided by big pharma organisations. Below is the wider manufacturing supply chain which constitutes various suppliers (lab equipment, chemicals etc.), R&D and discovery, production and delivery. Marketing, therefore, exists heavily in both B2C and B2B pharmaceutical environments to inform stakeholders of the options available to them.

2. Characteristics of the Market

The pharmaceutical market consists of a large degree of regulation and administrative oversight, complex payment systems as well as the involvement of multiple decision markers, which limits the nature of the marketing of pharmaceutical products and services. For the pharmaceutical organisations themselves, the importance of innovation cannot be overstated: New drugs provide gains to consumers (patients and payors) in the form of clinical benefits over existing treatments; generic drugs provide gains to consumers (patients and payors) in the form of lower costs. (Tepperman, 2009)

Marketers are required to always be aware of this. All of which leads to the importance of product differentiation - in both B2C and B2B sectors. Therapeutic substitution, prescribing patterns, manufacturing innovations, as well as the competition, intertwine to define this differentiation which marketers strive to achieve to make the product exchange. Every exchange requires that (1) there are two or more parties (2) interested in satisfying their unfulfilled desires, (3) have something of value to offer to each other, and (4) are capable of communication and delivery.

3. Keeping in Touch with the Market

The management of pharmaceutical marketing broadly entails keeping in touch with the changes within the market. This might include the analysis, planning and implementation of new marketing strategies to attract target audiences that invariably achieve organisation-wide objectives, such as marketing share, revenue or sales volume.

Just as patient preferences change, so does the consolidation, outsourcing, acquisitions and partnerships within the supply chain. It is, therefore, key that systems, cultures and marketing messages are integrated in order to capture value and make this known to target audiences. The same principles apply when external factors, such as the Coronavirus pandemic, disrupt the way in which markets - all of the stakeholders involved from the patients, HCPs, manufacturers and governments etc. - operate.

4. Pharmaceutical Market Research

The process of researching a pharmaceutical market or sub-market is a highly complex process. Defining its capacity, need, level of demand (and the ability to supply) and the motivations of the customer segments determine the marketing strategy, as well as budget, of a pharmaceutical product or service.

We've previously written a post on market research - A B2B Pharma Market Research Guide that goes into more depth than this management overview and provides guidance related to SWOT analysis, market intelligence, surveys and benchmarking within a methodical process. This process involves (1) problem and research objective definition, (2) research planning, (3) data collection, (4) data analysis, (5) data interpretation and finally, (6) reporting of findings. The basic components of a market mechanism is demand, the price and the offer of goods in the market - this is always a safe avenue to begin your pharmaceutical market research.

5. Product Life Cycle

Products and services sit centrally within the marketing plan or strategy; when there is no product/services marketing isn't required. Marketing has the ability to enhance a product or services image but effectively positioning it within a given market and communicating the benefits and satisfaction that follows a purchase. Such pharmaceutical products and services usually go through different stages, each stage being affected by different competitive conditions. These stages require different marketing strategies at different times if sales and profits are to be efficiently realised. Pharmaceutical marketers must identify the life cycle stages which their products and services sit within for effective pharmaceutical marketing management.

Introduction is the period, during which the initial market acceptance may be in doubt; it may be a period of slow growth. Profits are often absent because of high marketing and other expenses. The promotional elements during this stage revolves around different combinations of product, price and distribution factors. Survivors of the introduction stage generally enjoy a period of growth. During this period there is substantial profit improvement. The strategy in this stage takes the following shape: (a) product improvement - the addition of new features and models; (b) development of new market segments; (c) selective demand stimulation; and (d) price adjustments. During the next stage, maturity, there is rivalry for a mature market. Battling to retain the company's share, each marketer steps up promotion and perhaps grants price concessions. Finally, there is a decline period, which may be steep. Though sales and profits continue their downward trend, the declining product is not necessarily unprofitable as the competition may have been removed by this stage.

6. Product Positioning

As previously mentioned, differentiation is required to position a pharmaceutical marketing product, service or brand within the market, with the aim of receiving a favourable reception compared to the products of competitors. Effective market research will also indicate the segment of the market which the product and its positioning statement will likely succeed. Positioning indicates what the product stands for, what it is, and how the customers should evaluate it and the process can be determined in relation to a competitor, segment, category, quality or price.

7. Pricing Factors

So far, much of the factors in this post may not seem to relate to the day-to-day pharmaceutical marketer focused on preparing press releases, coordinating media plans with agencies as well as managing digital events. But strategic marketers will realise that each organisation, product/service and marketing plan does not operate within isolation, and, therefore, factors such as competitive pricing in relation to a marketing message is essential. Both internal and external factors will influence factors, such as marketing orientation, strategy, costs and product life cycle as well as competitive pricing factors - some of these factors are listed in the diagram below.

Although related to the practice of marketing management, pricing policy and strategy is set out at an organisation-wide level. The price policy is the complex of measures including determining of the price, extra charges and discounts, conditions of payment for the goods and services, management of the prices taking into account preferences and possibilities of consumers the maintenance of profit of the enterprise-manufacturer or the seller. Working out of a marketing price policy is preceded by the analysis of external and internal factors of its formation, in turn, as a part of the price policy research of consequences of changes of the price depending on a situation in the market (reaction of buyers and competitors, enterprise actions in reply to changes of the prices by competitors, etc.) should be provided.

8. Sales and Marketing Alignment

Pharmaceutical marketing will never exist in isolation and will mostly work hand-in-hand with sales departments, representatives of the products or HCPs. This is the case as the producer of pharmaceutical products rarely sells its products directly to the consumer - the product goes via the pharmacy, hospital, wholesalers, retailers or other intermediaries to get into the patient. Similarly, sales representatives of supply chain manufacturers are required for those organisations to buy and sell from each other. The very nature of the industry dictates that multiple decision markers are involved, meaning that marketing strategies must consider the use of sales (and other middle-men) to be successful.

Effective pharmaceutical marketing management requires marketing and sales (or any other intermediary) to be fully aligned and working towards the same commercial goals. See recent post on Closed-Loop Marketing in Pharma for more.

9. Marketing Communications

Along with the tasks of market research, pricing, positioning and marketing policy aforementioned, marketing involves the actions of pharmaceutical marketers to create a demand for goods and sales promotion via its marketing communications plan. The 7Ps Marketing Mix is the combination of elements used by a business to enable it to meet the needs and expectations of its customers. They combine to form the elements a marketing department need to review to promote the organisation successfully.

This would entail all of the customer-facing pharmaceutical marketing tactics that take this product to market and includes advertising, PR, branding, trade channels and other customer-facing experiences. The management of the marketing plan alone within the pharmaceutical sectors often involves an entire team of marketing-specific roles and specialities. Through various activities to generate demand and, above all, commercial marketing and advertising in the minds of potential customers created a positive image of the products and services and plays a major role in deciding on a purchase.

10. Data Analytics

The business and management textbooks of old will not have prepared the traditional pharmaceutical marketing manager to what would follow in the turn of the 21st century. Pharmaceutical marketing departments will have access to masses of data from marketing campaigns, from continually monitoring the market as well as the data gathered by other departments such as sales or customer service. All of which provides valuable insight into future marketing campaigns. The majority of this process will look at your own marketing metrics - such as website visitors, conversions and number of leads/sales generated but to be able to fully understand the the data you have you will need to analyse it in a number of ways. Data and analytics will play an important factor in the management of your marketing plan.

11. Control and Management

The fundamental aspect of successful marketing management is the control of the marketing plan. Control refers to the analytical work carried out on a day-to-day and month-by-month basis, where as a result, the marketing executives can determine new methods of marketing tactics, tools and management as the organisation optimises and adapts to its environment. Generally speaking, it provides an overview of what has not worked (so that those marketing initiatives can be discontinued) and what has worked (so that those marketing initiatives can be expanded).

Control of marketing includes the evaluation of the implementation of marketing strategies and implementing corrective actions to achieve their goals. The basic parameters of control are volume sales, profit margins and costs, consumer response on new products and services, compliance with the planned and actual results of industrial and commercial activities. Marketing control allows the company to determine the effectiveness of marketing opportunities, and as a management principle, it is hugely important for the success of the commercial activities of the pharmaceutical organisation. To health care providers

Marketing to health-care providers takes three main forms: activity by pharmaceutical sales representatives, provision of drug samples, and sponsoring continuing medical education (CME). The use of gifts, including pens and coffee mugs embossed with pharmaceutical product names, has been prohibited by PHRMA ethics guidelines since 2008. Of the 237,000 medical sites representing 680,000 physicians surveyed in SK&A's 2010 Physician Access survey, half said they prefer or require an appointment to see a rep (up from 38.5% preferring or requiring an appointment in 2008), while 23% won't see reps at all, according to the survey data. Practices owned by hospitals or health systems are tougher to get into than private practices, since appointments have to go through headquarters, the survey found. 13.3% of offices with just one or two doctors won't see representatives, compared with a no-see rate of 42% at offices with 10 or more doctors. The most accessible physicians for promotional purposes are allergists/immunologists – only 4.2% won't see reps at all – followed by orthopedic specialists (5.1%) and diabetes specialists

(7.6%). Diagnostic radiologists are the most rigid about allowing details – 92.1% won't see reps – followed by pathologists and neuroradiologists, at 92.1% and 91.8%, respectively.

E-detailing is widely used to reach "no see physicians"; approximately 23% of primary care physicians and 28% of specialists prefer computer-based e-detailing, according to survey findings reported in the 25 April 2011, edition of American Medical News (AMNews), published by the American Medical Association (AMA).

PhRMA Code

The Pharmaceutical Research and Manufacturers of America (PhRMA) released updates to its voluntary Code on Interactions with Healthcare Professionals on 10 July 2008. The new guidelines took effect in January 2009."

In addition to prohibiting small gifts and reminder items such as pens, notepads, staplers, clipboards, paperweights, pill boxes, etc., the revised Code:

Prohibits company sales representatives providing restaurant meals to healthcare professionals, but allows them to provide occasional modest meals in healthcare professionals' offices in conjunction with informational presentations"

Includes new provisions requiring companies to ensure their representatives are sufficiently trained about applicable laws, regulations, and industry codes of practice and ethics.

Provides that each company will state its intentions to abide by the Code and that company CEOs and compliance officers will certify each year that they have processes in place to comply.

Includes more detailed standards regarding the independence of continuing medical education.

Provides additional guidance and restrictions for speaking and consulting arrangements with healthcare professionals.

Free samples

Free samples have been shown to affect physician prescribing behavior. Physicians with access to free samples are more likely to prescribe brand name medication over equivalent generic medications. Other studies found that free samples decreased the likelihood that physicians would follow the standard of care practices.

Receiving pharmaceutical samples does not reduce prescription costs. Even after receiving samples, sample recipients remain disproportionately burdened by prescription costs.

It is argued that a benefit to free samples is the "try it before you buy it" approach. Free samples give immediate access to the medication and the patient can begin treatment right away. Also, it saves time from going to a pharmacy to get it filled before treatment begins. Since not all medications work for everyone, and many do not work the same way for each person, free samples allow patients to find which dose and brand of medication works best before having to spend money on a filled prescription at a pharmacy.

Continuing medical Education

Hours spent by physicians in industry-supported continuing medical education (CME) is greater than that from either medical schools or professional societies.

Pharmaceutical Representatives

Currently, there are approximately 81,000 pharmaceutical sales representatives in the United States pursuing some 830,000 pharmaceutical prescribers. A pharmaceutical representative will often try to see a given physician every few weeks. Representatives often have a call list of about 200–300 physicians with 120–180 targets that should be visited in 1–2 or 3 week cycle.

Because of the large size of the pharmaceutical sales force, the organization, management, and measurement of effectiveness of the sales force are significant business challenges. Management tasks are usually broken down into the areas of physician targeting, sales force size and structure, sales force optimization, call planning, and sales forces effectiveness. A few pharmaceutical companies have realized that training sales representatives on high science alone is not enough, especially when most products are similar in quality. Thus, training sales representatives on relationship selling techniques in addition to medical science and product knowledge, can make a difference in sales force effectiveness. Specialist physicians are relying more and more on specialty sales reps for product information, because they are more knowledgeable than primary care reps.

The United States has 81,000 pharmaceutical representatives or 1 for every 7.9 physicians. The number and persistence of pharmaceutical representatives has placed a burden on the time of physicians. "As the number of reps went up, the amount of time an average rep spent with doctors went down—so far down, that tactical scaling has spawned a strategic crisis. Physicians no longer spend much time with sales reps, nor do they see this as a serious problem."

Marketers must decide on the appropriate size of a sales force needed to sell a particular portfolio of drugs to the target market. Factors influencing this decision are the optimal reach (how many physicians to see) and frequency (how often to see them) for each individual physician, how many patients suffer from that disease state, how many sales representatives to devote to office and group practice and how many to devote to hospital accounts if needed. To aid this decision, customers are broken down into different classes according to their prescription behavior, patient population, their business potential, and event their personality traits.

Marketers attempt to identify the set of physicians most likely to prescribe a given drug. Historically, this was done by drug reps 'on the ground' using zip code sales and engaging in recon to figure out who the high prescribers were in a particular sales territory. However, in the mid-1990s the industry, through 3rd party prescribing data (e.g., Quintiles/IMS) switched to "script-tracking" technologies, measuring the number of total prescriptions (TRx) and new prescriptions (NRx) per week that each physician writes. This information is collected by commercial vendors. The physicians are then "deciled" into ten groups based on their writing patterns. Higher deciles are more aggressively targeted. Some pharmaceutical companies use additional information such as:

Profitability of a prescription (script),

Accessibility of the physician,

Tendency of the physician to use the pharmaceutical company's drugs,

Effect of managed care formularies on the ability of the physician to prescribe a drug,

The adoption sequence of the physician (that is, how readily the physician adopts new drugs in place of older treatments), and

The tendency of the physician to use a wide palette of drugs

Influence that physicians have on their colleagues.

Physicians are perhaps the most important component in sales. They write the prescriptions that determine which drugs will be used by people. Influencing the physician is the key to pharmaceutical sales. Historically, by a large pharmaceutical sales force. A medium-sized pharmaceutical company might have a sales force of 1000 representatives. The largest companies have tens of thousands of representatives around the world. Sales representatives called upon physicians regularly, providing clinical information, approved journal articles, and free drug samples. This is still the approach today; however, economic pressures on the industry are causing pharmaceutical companies to rethink the traditional sales process to physicians. The industry has seen a large scale adoption of Pharma CRM systems that works on laptops and more recently tablets. The new age pharmaceutical representative is armed with key data at his fingertips and tools to maximize the time spent with physicians.

Pharmaceutical Company Payments

Pharmaceutical and medical device companies have also paid physicians to use their drugs, which could affect how often a drug is prescribed. For example, one study that looked at physician payments and pimavanserin found that "extensive physician payments have been associated with increased pimavanserin prescription volume and Medicare expenditures."

More specifically, drug reps help to create a culture of gifting, or the "pharmaceutical gift exchange," where actual monetary transactions are rare. In reality, gifts, both large and small, ranging from cups of coffee to travel to medical conferences are exchanged on a routine basis with high prescribers in an effort to shift their obligations from patients to prescriptions and have proven effective.

Peer influence

Key opinion leaders

Key opinion leaders (KOL), or "thought leaders", are respected individuals, such as prominent medical school faculty, who influence physicians through their professional status. Pharmaceutical companies generally engage key opinion leaders early in the drug development process to provide advocacy and key marketing feedback. Some pharmaceutical companies identify key opinion leaders through direct inquiry of physicians (primary research). Recently, pharmaceutical companies have begun to use social network analysis to uncover thought leaders; because it does not introduce respondent bias, which is commonly found in primary research; it can identify and map out the entire scientific community for a disease state; and it has greater compliance with state and federal regulations; because physician prescribing patterns are not used to create the social network.

Alternatives to segmenting physicians purely on the basis of prescribing do exist, and marketers can call upon strategic partners who specialize in delineating which characteristics of true opinion leadership, a physician does or does not possess. Such analyses can help guide marketers in how to optimize KOL engagements as bona fide advisors to a brand, and can help shape clinical development and clinical data publication plans for instance, ultimately advancing patient care.

Colleagues

Physicians acquire information through informal contacts with their colleagues, including social events, professional affiliations, common hospital affiliations, and common medical school affiliations. Some pharmaceutical companies identify influential colleagues through commercially available prescription writing and patient level data. Doctor dinner meetings are an effective way for physicians to acquire educational information from respected peers and to influence the so called "no-see" physicians - those that are reluctant to engage directly with pharmaceutical reps through detailing but may come to a dinner program where a local or national expert is talking. These meetings are sponsored by some pharmaceutical companies.

Journal Articles and Technical Documentation

Recent legal cases and US congressional hearings have provided access to pharmaceutical industry documents revealing new marketing strategies for drugs. Activities once considered independent of promotional intent, including continuing medical education and medical research, are used, including paying to publish articles about promoted drugs for the medical literature, and alleged suppression of unfavorable study results.

Private and Public Insurers

Public and private insurers affect the writing of prescriptions by physicians through formularies that restrict the number and types of drugs that the insurer will cover. Not only can the insurer affect drug sales by including or excluding a particular drug from a formulary, they can affect sales by tiering, or placing bureaucratic hurdles to prescribing certain drugs. In January 2006, the United States instituted a new public prescription drug plan through its Medicare program. Known as Medicare Part D, this program engages private insurers to negotiate with pharmaceutical companies for the placement of drugs on tiered formularies.

To consumers

Only two countries as of 2008 allow direct to consumer advertising (DTCA): the United States and New Zealand. Since the late 1970s, DTCA of prescription drugs has become important in the United States. It takes two main forms: the promotion or creation of a disease out of a non-pathologic physical condition or the promotion of a medication. The rhetorical objective of direct-to-consumer advertising is to directly influence the patient-physician dialogue. Many patients will inquire about, or even demand a medication they have seen advertised on television. In the United States, recent years have seen an increase in mass media advertisements for pharmaceuticals. Expenditures on direct-to-users advertising almost quadrupled in the seven years between 1997 and 2005 since the FDA changed the guidelines, from $1.1 billion in 1997 to more than $4.2 billion in 2005, a 19.6% annual increase, according to the United States Government Accountability Office, 2006).

The mass marketing to users of pharmaceuticals is banned in over 30 industrialized nations, but not in the US and New Zealand, which is considering a ban. Some feel it is better to leave the decision wholly in the hands of medical professionals; others feel that users education and participation in health is useful, but users need independent, comparative information about drugs (not promotional information). For these reasons, most countries impose limits on pharmaceutical mass marketing that are not placed on the marketing of other products. In some areas it is required that ads for drugs include a list of possible side effects, so that users are informed of both facets of a medicine. Canada's limitations on pharmaceutical advertising ensure that commercials that mention the name of a product cannot in any way describe what it does. Commercials that mention a medical problem cannot also mention the name of the product for sale; at most, they can direct the viewer to a website or telephone number operated by the pharmaceutical company.

Reynold Spector has provided examples of how positive and negative hype can affect perceptions of pharmaceuticals using examples of certain cancer drugs, such as Avastin and Opdivo, in the former case and statins in the latter.

Drug coupons

In the United States, pharmaceutical companies often provide drug coupons to consumers to help offset the copayments charged by health insurers for prescription medication. These coupons are generally used to promote medications that compete with non-preferred products and cheaper, generic alternatives by reducing or eliminating the extra out-of-pocket costs that an insurers typically charge a patient for a non-preferred drug product.

Economics

Pharmaceutical company spending on marketing exceeds that spent on research. In 2004 in Canada $1.7 billion a year was spent marketing drugs to physicians and in the United States $21 billion were spent in 2002. In 2005 money spent on pharmaceutical marketing in the United States was estimated at $29.9 billion with one estimate as high as $57 billion. When the US number are broken down 56% was free samples, 25% was detailing of physicians, 12.5% was direct to users advertising, 4% on hospital detailing, and 2% on journal ads. In the United States approximately $20 billion could be saved if generics were used instead of equivalent brand name products.

Although pharmaceutical companies have made large investments in marketing their products, overall promotional spending has been decreasing over the last few years, and declined by 10 percent from 2009 to 2010. Pharmaceutical companies are cutting back mostly in detailing and sampling, while spending in mailings and print advertising grew since last year.

Evolution of Marketing

The emergence of new media and technologies in recent years is quickly changing the pharmaceutical marketing landscape in the United States. Both physicians and users are increasing their reliance on the Internet as a source of health and medical information, prompting pharmaceutical marketers to look at digital channels for opportunities to reach their target audiences.

In 2008, 84% of U.S. physicians used the Internet and other technologies to access pharmaceutical, biotech or medical device information—a 20% increase from 2004. At the same time, sales reps are finding it more difficult to get time with doctors for in-person details. Pharmaceutical companies are exploring online marketing as an alternative way to reach physicians. Emerging e-promotional activities include live video detailing, online events, electronic sampling, and physician customer service portals such as PV Updates, MDLinx, Aptus Health (former Physicians Interactive), and Epocrates.

Direct-to-users marketers are also recognizing the need to shift to digital channels as audiences become more fragmented and the number of access points for news, entertainment and information multiplies. Standard television, radio and print direct-to-users (DTC) advertisements are less relevant than in the past, and companies are beginning to focus more on digital marketing efforts like product websites, online display advertising, search engine marketing, social media campaigns, place-based media and mobile advertising to reach the over 145 million U.S. adults online for health information.

In 2010, the FDA's Division of Drug Marketing, Advertising and Communications issued a warning letter concerning two unbranded consumer targeted Web sites sponsored by Novartis Pharmaceuticals Corporation as the websites promoted a drug for an unapproved use, the websites failed to disclose the risks associated with the use of the drug and made unsubstantiated dosing claims.

Orientations

A marketing orientation has been defined as a "philosophy of business management." or "a corporate state of mind" or as an "organisation[al] culture" Although scholars continue to debate the precise nature of specific orientations that inform marketing practice, the most commonly cited orientations are as follows:

Product

A firm employing a product orientation is mainly concerned with the quality of its own product. A product orientation is based on the assumption that, all things being equal, consumers will purchase products of a superior quality. The approach is most effective when the firm has deep insights into customers and their needs and desires derived from research and (or) intuition and understands consumers' quality expectations and price they are willing to pay. For example, Sony Walkman and Apple iPod were innovative product designs that addressed consumers' unmet needs. Although the product orientation has largely been supplanted by the marketing orientation, firms practising a product orientation can still be found in haute couture and in arts marketing.

Sales

A firm using a sales orientation focuses primarily on the selling/promotion of the firm's existing products, rather than determining new or unmet consumer needs or desires. Consequently, this entails simply selling existing products, using promotion and direct sales techniques to attain the highest sales possible. The sales orientation "is typically practised with unsought goods." One study found that industrial companies are more likely to hold a sales orientation than consumer goods companies. The approach may also suit scenarios in which a firm holds dead stock, or otherwise sells a product that is in high demand, with little likelihood of changes in consumer tastes diminishing demand. A 2011 meta analyses has found that the factors with the greatest impact on sales performance are a salesperson's sales related knowledge (knowledge of market segments, sales presentation skills, conflict resolution, and products), degree of adaptiveness (changing behaviour based on the aforementioned knowledge), role clarity (salesperson's role is to expressly to sell), cognitive aptitude (intelligence) and work engagement (motivation and interest in a sales role).

Production

A firm focusing on a production orientation specializes in producing as much as possible of a given product or service in order to achieve economies of scale or economies of scope. A production orientation may be deployed when a high demand for a product or service exists, coupled with certainty that consumer tastes and preferences remain relatively constant (similar to the sales orientation). The so-called production era is thought to have dominated marketing practice from the 1860s to the 1930s, but other theorists argue that evidence of the production orientation can still be found in some companies or industries. Specifically Kotler and Armstrong note that the production philosophy is "one of the oldest philosophies that guides sellers... [and] is still useful in some situations."

Marketing

The marketing orientation is perhaps the most common orientation used in contemporary marketing. It is a customer-centric approach that involves a firm basing its marketing program around products that suit new consumer tastes. Firms adopting a marketing orientation typically engage in extensive market research to gauge consumer desires, use R&D to develop a product attuned to the revealed information, and then utilize promotion techniques to ensure consumers are aware of the product's existence and the benefits it can deliver. Scales designed to measure a firm's overall market orientation have been developed and found to be relatively robust in a variety of contexts.

The marketing orientation often has three prime facets, which are:

Customer orientation: A firm in the market economy can survive by producing goods that persons are willing and able to buy. Consequently, ascertaining consumer demand is vital for a firm's future viability and even existence as a going concern.

Organizational orientation: In this sense, a firm's marketing department is often seen as of prime importance within the functional level of an organization. Information from an organization's marketing department would be used to guide the actions of other department's within the firm. As an example, a marketing department could ascertain (via marketing research) that consumers desired a new type of product, or a new usage for an existing product. With this in mind, the marketing department would inform the R&D department to create a prototype of a product/service based on consumers' new desires.

The production department would then start to manufacture the product, while the marketing department would focus on the promotion, distribution, pricing, etc. of the product. Additionally, a firm's finance department would be consulted, with respect to securing appropriate funding for the development, production and promotion of the product. Inter-departmental conflicts may occur, should a firm adhere to the marketing orientation. Production may oppose the installation, support and servicing of new capital stock, which may be needed to manufacture a new product. Finance may oppose the required capital expenditure, since it could undermine a healthy cash flow for the organization.

Mutually beneficial exchange: In a transaction in the market economy, a firm gains revenue, which thus leads to more profits/market share/sales. A consumer on the other hand gains the satisfaction of a need/want, utility, reliability and value for money from the purchase of a product or service. As no-one has to buy goods from any one supplier in the market economy, firms must entice consumers to buy goods with contemporary marketing ideals.

Regulation and Fraud

European Union

In the European Union, marketing of pharmaceuticals is regulated by EU (formerly EEC) Directive 92/28/EEC. Among other things, it requires member states to prohibit off-label marketing, and direct-to-consumer marketing of prescription-only medications.

United States

In the United States, marketing and distribution of pharmaceuticals is regulated by the Federal Food, Drug, and Cosmetic Act and the Prescription Drug Marketing Act, respectively. Food and Drug Administration (FDA) regulations require all prescription drug promotion to be truthful and not misleading, based on "substantial evidence or substantial clinical experience", to provide a "fair balance" between the risks and benefits of the promoted drug, and to maintain consistency with labeling approved by the FDA. The FDA Office of Prescription Drug Promotion enforces these requirements.

In the 1990s, antipsychotics were "still seen as treatments for the most serious mental illnesses, like hallucinatory schizophrenia, and recast them for much broader uses". Drugs such as Abilify and Geodon were given to a broad range of patients, from preschoolers to octogenarians. In 2010, more than a half-million youths took antipsychotic drugs, and one-quarter of nursing-home residents have used them. Yet the government warns that the drugs may be fatal to some older patients and have unknown effects on children.

Every major company selling the drugs—Bristol-Myers Squibb, Eli Lilly, Pfizer, AstraZeneca, and Johnson & Johnson—has either settled recent government cases, under the False Claims Act, for hundreds of millions of dollars or is currently under investigation for possible health care fraud. Following charges of illegal marketing, two of the settlements in 2009 set records for the largest criminal fines ever imposed on corporations. One involved Eli Lilly's antipsychotic Zyprexa, and the other involved Bextra. In the Bextra case, the government also charged Pfizer with illegally marketing another antipsychotic, Geodon; Pfizer settled that part of the claim for $301 million, without admitting any wrongdoing.

SOCIETAL MARKETING

A number of scholars and practitioners have argued that marketers have a greater social responsibility than simply satisfying customers and providing them with superior value. Instead, marketing activities should strive to benefit society's overall well-being. Marketing organisations that have embraced the societal marketing concept typically identify key stakeholder groups such as employees, customers, and local communities. They should consider the impact of their activities on all stakeholders. Companies that adopt a societal marketing perspective typically practice triple bottom line reporting whereby they publish social impact and environmental impact reports alongside financial performance reports. Sustainable marketing or green marketing is an extension of societal marketing.

The Marketing mix (the 4 Ps)

As a mnemonic for 'product', 'price', 'place' and 'promotion', the four Ps are often referred to as the marketing mix or the marketing program, represent the basic tools which marketers can use to bring their products or services to market. They are the foundation of managerial marketing and the marketing plan typically devotes a section to each of these Ps.

Origins

During the 1940s, the discipline of marketing was in transition. Interest in the functional school of thought, which was primarily concerned with mapping the functions of marketing was waning while the managerial school of thought, which focussed on the problems and challenges confronting marketers was gaining ground. The concept of marketers as "mixers of ingredients," was first introduced by James Culliton, a Professor at Harvard Business School. At this time theorists began to develop checklists of the elements that made up the marketing mix, however, there was little agreement as to what should be included in the list. Many scholars and practitioners relied on lengthy classifications of factors that needed to be considered to understand consumer responses. Neil Borden developed a complicated model in the late 1940s, based upon at least twelve different factors.

Inspired by the idea of marketers as mixers of ingredients, Neil Borden one of Culliton's colleagues at Harvard, coined the phrase the marketing mix and used it wherever possible. According to Borden's own account, he used the term, 'marketing mix' consistently from the late 1940s. For instance, he is on record as having used the term, 'marketing mix,' in his presidential address given to the American Marketing Association in 1953. In the mid-1960s, Borden published a retrospective article detailing the early history of the marketing mix in which he claims that he was inspired by Culliton's idea of 'mixers', and credits himself with coining the term, 'marketing mix'. Borden's continued and consistent use of the phrase, "marketing mix," contributed to the process of popularising the concept throughout the 1940s and 50s.

The "marketing mix" gained widespread acceptance with the publication, in 1960, of E. Jerome McCarthy's text, Basic Marketing: A Managerial Approach which outlined the ingredients in the mix as the memorable 4 Ps, namely product, price, place and promotion. The marketing mix is based upon four controllable variables that a company manages in its effort to satisfy the corporation's objectives as well as the needs and wants of a target market. Once there is understanding of the target market's interests, marketers develop tactics, using the 4Ps, to encourage buyers to purchase product. The successful use of the model is predicated upon the degree to which the target market's needs and wants have been understood, and the extent to which marketers have developed and correctly deployed the tactics. Today, the marketing mix or marketing program is understood to refer to the "set of marketing tools that the firm uses to pursue its marketing objectives in the target market".

Brief Outline

The traditional marketing mix refers to four broad levels of marketing decision, namely: product, price, promotion, and place.

Product

The product aspects of marketing deal with the specifications of the actual goods or services, and how it relates to the end-user's needs and wants. The product element consists of product design, new product innovation, branding, packaging, labelling. The scope of a product generally includes supporting elements such as warranties, guarantees, and support. Branding, a key aspect of the product management, refers to the various methods of communicating a brand identity for the product, brand, or company.

Pricing

This refers to the process of setting a price for a product, including discounts. The price need not be monetary; it can simply be what is exchanged for the product or services, e.g. time, energy, or attention or any sacrifices consumers make in order to acquire a product or service. The price is the cost that a consumer pays for a product—monetary or not. Methods of setting prices are in the domain of pricing science.

Place (Distribution)

This refers to how the product gets to the customer; the distribution channels and intermediaries such as wholesalers and retailers who enable customers to access products or services in a convenient manner. This third P has also sometimes been called Place, referring to the channel by which a product or service is sold (e.g. online vs. retail), which geographic region or industry, to which segment (young adults, families, business people), etc. also referring to how the environment in which the product is sold in can affect sales.

Promotion

This includes all aspects of marketing communications; advertising, sales promotion, including promotional education, public relations, personal selling, product placement, branded entertainment, event marketing, trade shows and exhibitions.

Criticisms

Morgan, in Riding the Waves of Change (Jossey-Bass, 1988), suggests that one of the greatest limitations of the 4 Ps approach "is that it unconsciously emphasizes the inside–out view (looking from the company outwards), whereas the essence of marketing should be the outside–in approach". An inside-out approach is the traditional planning approach where the organisation identifies its desired goals and objectives which are often based around what has always been done. Marketing's task then becomes one of "selling" the organisation's products and messages to the "outside" or external stakeholders. In contrast, an outside-in approach first seeks to understand the needs and wants of the consumer.

From a model-building perspective, the 4 Ps has attracted a number of criticisms. Well-designed models should exhibit clearly defined categories that are mutually exclusive, with no overlap. Yet, the 4 Ps model has extensive overlapping problems. Some of the Ps are only defined in vague terms. Several authors stress the hybrid nature of the fourth P, mentioning the presence of two important dimensions, "communication" (general and informative communications such as public relations and corporate communications) and "promotion" (persuasive communications such as advertising and direct selling). Certain marketing activities, such as personal selling, may be classified as either promotion or as part of the place (i.e. distribution) element. Some pricing tactics such as promotional pricing can be classified as price variables or promotional variables and therefore also exhibit some overlap.

Other important criticisms include that the marketing mix lacks a strategic framework and is therefore unfit to be a planning instrument, particularly when uncontrollable, external elements are an important aspect of the marketing environment.

Modifications and Extensions

To overcome the deficiencies of the 4 P model, some authors have suggested extensions or modifications to the original model. Extensions of the four P's include "people", "process", and "physical evidence" and are often applied in the case of services marketing Other extensions have been found necessary in retail marketing, industrial marketing and internet marketing:

- Industrial marketing or B2B marketing needs to account for the long term contractual agreements that are typical in supply chain transactions. Relationship marketingattempts to do this by looking at marketing from a long term relationship perspective rather than individual transactions.

- Services marketing needs to account for the unique characteristics of services (i.e. intangibility, perishability, heterogeneity and the inseparability of production and consumption). In order to recognize the special challenges involved in selling services, as opposed to goods, some authors advocate extending the model to 7 Ps for service industries by adding; Process – the way in which orders are handled, customers are satisfied and the service is delivered; Physical Evidence – is tangible evidence with which customers interact and with the potential to impact on the customer's service experience; People – service personnel and other customers with whom customers interact and form part of the overall service experience.

Expanded Marketing mix for Retail

- Retail marketing needs to account for the unique facets of retail stores. A number of authors have argued for the inclusion of two new Ps, namely, Personnel and Presentation since these contribute to the customer's unique retail experience and are the principal basis for retail differentiation. Some scholars also recommend adding Retail Format (i.e. retail formula) since it contributes to customer expectations. The modified retail marketing mix is often called the 6 Ps of retailing.
- Internet marketing presents both marketing practitioners and scholars with special challenges including: customer empowerment, new communication modes, real-time interactivity, access to global markets, high levels of market transparency and difficulty maintaining competitive advantages. While some scholars argue for an expanded marketing mix for internet marketing, most argue that entirely new models are required.
- Some authors cite a further P – Packaging – this is thought by many to be part of Product, but in certain markets (Japan, China for example) and with certain products (perfume, cosmetics) the packaging of a product has a greater importance – maybe even than the product itself.

ENVIRONMENT

The term "marketing environment" relates to all of the factors (whether internal, external, direct or indirect) that affect a firm's marketing decision-making/planning. A firm's marketing environment consists of three main areas, which are:

- The macro-environment, over which a firm holds little control
- The micro-environment, over which a firm holds a greater amount (though not necessarily total) control

- The internal environment, which includes the factors inside of the company itself

Macro

A firm's marketing macro-environment consists of a variety of external factors that manifest on a large (or macro) scale. These are typically economic, social, political or technological phenomena. A common method of assessing a firm's macro-environment is via a PESTLE (Political, Economic, Social, Technological, Legal, Ecological) analysis. Within a PESTLE analysis, a firm would analyze national political issues, culture and climate, key macroeconomic conditions, health and indicators (such as economic growth, inflation, unemployment, etc.), social trends/attitudes, and the nature of technology's impact on its society and the business processes within the society.

Micro

A firm's micro-environment comprises factors pertinent to the firm itself, or stakeholders closely connected with the firm or company.

A firm's micro-environment typically spans:

- Customers/consumers
- Employees
- Suppliers
- The Media

By contrast to the macro-environment, an organization holds a greater degree of control over these factors.

Internal

A firms internal environment consists of factors inside of the actual company. These are factors controlled by the firm and they affect the relationship that a firm has with its customers. These include factors such as:

- Labor
- Inventory
- Company Policy
- Logistics
- Budget
- Capital Assets

Research

Marketing research is a systematic process of analyzing data which involves conducting research to support marketing activities, and the statistical interpretation of data into information. This information is then used by managers to plan marketing activities, gauge the nature of a firm's marketing environment and to attain information from suppliers. A distinction should be made between marketing research and market research. Market research pertains to research in a given market. As an example, a firm may conduct research in a target market, after selecting a suitable market segment. In contrast, marketing research relates to all research conducted within marketing. Market research is a subset of marketing research.

Marketing researchers use statistical methods (such as quantitative research, qualitative research, hypothesis tests, Chi-square tests, linear regression, correlation coefficients, frequency distributions, Poisson and binomial distributions, etc.) to interpret their findings and convert data into information.

Research process

Marketing research spans a number of stages, including:

- Define the problem
- Develop a research plan
- Collect the data
- Interpret data into information
- Disseminate information formally in the form of a report

Segmentation

Market segmentation consists of taking the total heterogeneous market for a product and dividing it into several sub-markets or segments, each of which tends to be homogeneous in all significant aspects.

PURPOSES

Market segmentation is conducted for two main purposes, including:

- A better allocation of a firm's finite resources
- To better serve the more diversified tastes of contemporary consumers

A firm only possesses a certain amount of resources. Accordingly, it must make choices (and appreciate the related costs) in servicing specific groups of consumers.

Moreover, with more diversity in the tastes of modern consumers, firms are noting the benefit of servicing a multiplicity of new markets.

Overview

Market segmentation can be defined in terms of the STP acronym, meaning Segment, Target, Position.

Segment

Segmentation involves the initial splitting up of consumers into persons of like needs/wants/tastes.

Four commonly used criteria are used for segmentation, which include:

- Geographical (a country, region, city, town, etc.)

- Psychographic (e.g. personality traits or lifestyle traits which influence consumer behaviour)
- Demographic (e.g. age, gender, socio-economic class, education, etc.)
- Behavioural (e.g. brand loyalty, usage rate, etc.)

Target

Once a segment has been identified, a firm must ascertain whether the segment is beneficial for them to service.

The DAMP acronym (meaning Discernable, Accessible, Measurable and Profitable) are used as criteria to gauge the viability of a target market. The elements of DAMP are:

- Discernable – how a segment can be differentiated from other segments.
- Accessible – how a segment can be accessed via Marketing Communications produced by a firm
- Measurable – can the segment be quantified and its size determined?
- Profitable – can a sufficient return on investment be attained from a segment's servicing?

The next step in the targeting process is the level of differentiation involved in a segment serving. Three modes of differentiation exist, which are commonly applied by firms. These are:

- Undifferentiated – where a company produces a like product for all of a market segment
- Differentiated – in which a firm produced slight modifications of a product within a segment
- Niche – in which an organisation forges a product to satisfy a specialised target market

Position

Positioning concerns how to position a product in the minds of consumers and inform what attributes differentiate it from the competitor's products.

A firm often performs this by producing a perceptual map, which denotes similar products produced in the same industry according to how consumers perceive their price and quality. From a product's placing on the map, a firm would tailor its marketing communications to suit meld with the product's perception among consumers, and its position among competitors' offering.

Communications

Marketing communications is an audience-centered activity designed to engage audiences and promote responses. It is defined by actions a firm takes to communicate with end-users, consumers, and external parties.

Marketing communications encompass four distinct subsets, which are:

Personal Sales

Female beer sellers warn the photographer that he also has to buy some, Tireli market, Mali 1989

Oral presentation given by a salesperson who approaches individuals or a group of potential customers:

- Live, interactive relationship
- Personal interest
- Attention and response
- Interesting presentation
- Clear and thorough.

Sales Promotion

Short-term incentives to encourage buying of products:

- Instant appeal
- Anxiety to sell

An example is coupons or a sale. People are given an incentive to buy, but this does not build customer loyalty or encourage future repeat buys. A major drawback of sales promotion is that it is easily copied by competition. It cannot be used as a sustainable source of differentiation.

Public Relations

Public relations (or PR, as an acronym) is the use of media tools by a firm in order to promote goodwill from an organization to a target market segment, or other consumers of a firm's good/service. PR stems from the fact that a firm cannot seek to antagonize or inflame its market base, due to incurring a lessened demand for its good/service. Organizations undertake PR in order to assure consumers, and to forestall negative perceptions towards it.

PR can span:

- Interviews
- Speeches/Presentations
- Corporate literature, such as financial statements, brochures, etc.

Publicity

Publicity involves attaining space in media, without having to pay directly for such coverage. As an example, an organization may have the launch of a new product covered by a newspaper or TV news segment. This benefits the firm in question since it is making consumers aware of its product, without necessarily paying a newspaper or television station to cover the event.

Advertising

Advertising occurs when a firm directly pays a media channel to publicize its product. Common examples of this include TV and radio adverts, billboards, branding, sponsorship, etc.

Mix

Marketing communications mix is used to reach, engage, provoke audience-centered conversations. It consists of 5 tools, which are 1)Advertising, 2)Sales & Promotion, 3)Public Relations, 4)Direct Marketing and 5)Personal Selling. The types of messages that are enhanced can be 1)Informational, 2)Emotional, 3)User-generated, or/and 4)Brand content. The last main component of MC mix is Media, which corresponds to the channel used to send the message. Media is divided into 3 categories, and these are media by 1) Form, 2) Source and 3) Functionality.

Planning

The area of marketing planning involves forging a plan for a firm's marketing activities. A marketing plan can also pertain to a specific product, as well as to an organisation's overall marketing strategy.

Generally speaking, an organisation's marketing planning process is derived from its overall business strategy. Thus, when top management are devising the firm's strategic direction/mission, the intended marketing activities are incorporated into this plan.

Process

Within the overall strategic marketing plan, the stages of the process are listed as thus:

- Mission Statement
- Corporate Objectives
- Marketing Audit
- SWOT (Strengths, Weaknesses, Opportunities, Threats) analysis
- Assumptions arising from the Audit and SWOT analysis
- Marketing objectives derived from the assumptions
- An estimation of the expected results of the objectives
- Identification of alternative plans/mixes
- Budgeting for the marketing plan
- A first-year implementation program.

Levels of marketing objectives within an organization

As stated previously, the senior management of a firm would formulate a general business strategy for a firm. However, this general business strategy would be interpreted and implemented in different contexts throughout the firm.

Corporate

Corporate marketing objectives are typically broad-based in nature, and pertain to the general vision of the firm in the short, medium or long-term.

As an example, if one pictures a group of companies (or a conglomerate), top management may state that sales for the group should increase by 25% over a ten-year period.

Strategic Business Unit

A strategic business unit (SBU) is a subsidiary within a firm, which participates within a given market/industry. The SBU would embrace the corporate strategy, and attune it to its own particular industry. For instance, an SBU may partake in the sports goods industry. It thus would ascertain how it would attain additional sales of sports goods, in order to satisfy the overall business strategy.

Functional

The functional level relates to departments within the SBUs, such as marketing, finance, HR, production, etc. The functional level would adopt the SBU's strategy and determine how to accomplish the SBU's own objectives in its market.

To use the example of the sports goods industry again, the marketing department would draw up marketing plans, strategies and communications to help the SBU achieve its marketing aims.

Product Life Cycle

Further information: Product life-cycle management (marketing)

The product life cycle (PLC) is a tool used by marketing managers to gauge the progress of a product, especially relating to sales or revenue accrued over time. The PLC is based on a few key assumptions, including:

- A given product would possess introduction, growth, maturity, and decline stage
- No product lasts perpetually on the market
- A firm must employ differing strategies, according to where a product is on the PLC

Introduction

In this stage, a product is launched onto the market. To stimulate growth of sales/revenue, use of advertising may be high, in order to heighten awareness of the product in question.

Growth

The product's sales/revenue is increasing, which may stimulate more marketing communications to sustain sales. More entrants enter into the market, to reap the apparent high profits that the industry is producing.

Maturity

A product's sales start to level off, and an increasing number of entrants to a market produce price falls for the product. Firms may use sales promotions to raise sales.

Decline

Demand for a good begins to taper off, and the firm may opt to discontinue manufacture of the product. This is so, if revenue for the product comes from efficiency savings in production, over actual sales of a good/service. However, if a product services a niche market, or is complementary to another product, it may continue manufacture of the product, despite a low level of sales/revenue being accrued.

CUSTOMER FOCUS

Many companies today have a customer focus (or market orientation). This implies that the company focuses its activities and products on consumer demands. Generally there are three ways of doing this: the customer-driven approach, the sense of identifying market changes and the product innovation approach.

In the consumer-driven approach, consumer wants are the drivers of all strategic marketing decisions. No strategy is pursued until it passes the test of consumer research. Every aspect of a market offering, including the nature of the product itself, is driven by the needs of potential consumers. The starting point is always the consumer. The rationale for this approach is that there is no point spending R&D funds developing products that people will not buy. History attests to many products that were commercial failures in spite of being technological breakthroughs.

A formal approach to this customer-focused marketing is known as SIVA (Solution, Information, Value, Access). This system is basically the four Ps renamed and reworded to provide a customer focus.

The SIVA Model provides a demand/customer centric version alternative to the well-known 4Ps supply side model (product, price, place, promotion) of marketing management.

Product Focus

In a product innovation approach, the company pursues product innovation, then tries to develop a market for the product. Product innovation drives the process and marketing research is conducted primarily to ensure that profitable market segment(s) exist for the innovation. The rationale is that customers may not know what options will be available to them in the future so we should not expect them to tell us what they will buy in the future. However, marketers can aggressively over-pursue product innovation and try to overcapitalize on a niche. When pursuing a product innovation approach, marketers must ensure that they have a varied and multi-tiered approach to product innovation. It is claimed that if Thomas Edison depended on marketing research he would have produced larger candles rather than inventing light bulbs. Many firms, such as research and development focused companies, successfully focus on product innovation. Many purists doubt whether this is really a form of marketing orientation at all, because of the ex post status of consumer research. Some even question whether it is marketing.

- An emerging area of study and practice concerns internal marketing, or how employees are trained and managed to deliver the brand in a way that positively impacts the acquisition and retention of customers (employer branding).
- Diffusion of innovations research explores how and why people adopt new products, services and ideas.
- A relatively new form of marketing uses the Internet and is called Internet marketing or more generally e-marketing, affiliate marketing, desktop advertising or online marketing. It tries to perfect the segmentation strategy used in traditional marketing. It targets its audience more precisely, and is sometimes called personalized marketing or one-to-one marketing.
- With consumers' eroding attention span and willingness to give time to advertising messages, marketers are turning to forms of permission marketing such as branded content, custom media and reality marketing.
- The use of herd behavior in marketing.

The Economist reported a recent conference in Rome on the subject of the simulation of adaptive human behavior. It shared mechanisms to increase impulse buying and get people "to buy more by playing on the herd instinct." The basic idea is that people will buy more of products that are seen to be popular, and several feedback mechanisms to get product popularity information to consumers are mentioned, including smart-cart technology and the use of Radio Frequency Identification Tag technology. A "swarm-moves" model was introduced by a Florida Institute of Technology researcher, which is appealing to supermarkets because it can "increase sales without the need to give people discounts."

Marketing is also used to promote business' products and is a great way to promote the business.

Other recent studies on the "power of social influence" include an "artificial music market in which some 14,000 people downloaded previously unknown songs" (Columbia University, New York); a Japanese chain of convenience stores which orders its products based on "sales data from department stores and research companies;" a Massachusetts company exploiting knowledge of social networking to improve sales; and online retailers who are increasingly informing consumers about "which products are popular with like-minded consumers" (e.g., Amazon, eBay).

MARKETING MANAGEMENT

Structure

Marketing management employs tools from economics and competitive strategy to analyze the industry context in which the firm operates. These include Porter's five forces, analysis of strategic groups of competitors, value chain analysis and others.

In competitor analysis, marketers build detailed profiles of each competitor in the market, focusing on their relative competitive strengths and weaknesses using SWOT analysis. Marketing managers will examine each competitor's cost structure, sources of profits, resources and competencies, competitive positioning and product differentiation, degree of vertical integration, historical responses to industry developments, and other factors.

Marketing management often conduct market research and marketing research to perform marketing analysis. Marketers employ a variety of techniques to conduct market research, but some of the more common include:

- Qualitative marketing research, such as focus groups and various types of interviews
- Quantitative marketing research, such as statistical surveys
- Experimental techniques such as test markets
- Observational techniques such as ethnographic (on-site) observation

Marketing managers may also design and oversee various environmental scanning and competitive intelligence processes to help identify trends and inform the company's marketing analysis.

Brand Audit

A brand audit is a thorough examination of a brand's current position in an industry compared to its competitors and the examination of its effectiveness. When it comes to brand auditing, six questions should be carefully examined and assessed:

1. how well the business' current brand strategy is working,
2. what the company's established resource strengths and weaknesses are,
3. what its external opportunities and threats are,
4. how competitive the business' prices and costs are,
5. how strong the business' competitive position in comparison to its competitors is, and
6. what strategic issues are facing the business.

When a business is conducting a brand audit, the goal is to uncover business' resource strengths, deficiencies, best market opportunities, outside threats, future profitability, and its competitive standing in comparison to existing competitors. A brand audit establishes the strategic elements needed to improve brand position and competitive capabilities within the industry. Once a brand is audited, any business that ends up with a strong financial performance and market position is more likely than not to have a properly conceived and effectively executed brand strategy.

A brand audit examines whether a business' share of the market is increasing, decreasing, or stable. It determines if the company's margin of profit is improving, decreasing, and how much it is in comparison to the profit margin of established competitors. Additionally, a brand audit investigates trends in a business' net profits, the return on existing investments, and its established economic value. It determines whether or not the business' entire financial strength and credit rating is improving or getting worse. This kind of audit also assesses a business' image and reputation with its customers. Furthermore, a brand audit seeks to determine whether or not a business is perceived as an industry leader in technology, offering product or service innovations, along with exceptional customer service, among other relevant issues that customers use to decide on a brand of preference.

A brand audit usually focuses on a business' strengths and resource capabilities because these are the elements that enhance its competitiveness. A business' competitive strengths can exist in several forms. Some of these forms include skilled or pertinent expertise, valuable physical assets, valuable human assets, valuable organizational assets, valuable intangible assets, competitive capabilities, achievements and attributes that position the business into a competitive advantage, and alliances or cooperative ventures.

The basic concept of a brand audit is to determine whether a business' resource strengths are competitive assets or competitive liabilities. This type of audit seeks to ensure that a business maintains a distinctive competence that allows it to build and reinforce its competitive advantage. What's more, a successful brand audit seeks to establish what a business capitalizes on best, its level of expertise, resource strengths, and strongest competitive capabilities, while aiming to identify a business' position and future performance.

Marketing Strategy

Two customer segments are often selected as targets because they score highly on two dimensions:

1. The segment is attractive to serve because it is large, growing, makes frequent purchases, is not price sensitive (i.e. is willing to pay high prices), or other factors; and
2. The company has the resources and capabilities to compete for the segment's business, can meet their needs better than the competition, and can do so profitably.

A commonly cited definition of marketing is simply "meeting needs profitably".

The implication of selecting target segments is that the business will subsequently allocate more resources to acquire and retain customers in the target segment(s) than it will for other, non-targeted customers. In some cases, the firm may go so far as to turn away customers who are not in its target segment.The doorman at a swanky nightclub, for example, may deny entry to unfashionably dressed individuals because the business has made a strategic decision to target the "high fashion" segment of nightclub patrons.

In conjunction with targeting decisions, marketing managers will identify the desired positioning they want the company, product, or brand to occupy in the target customer's mind. This positioning is often an encapsulation of a key benefit the company's product or service offers that is differentiated and superior to the benefits offered by competitive products.For example, Volvo has traditionally positioned its products in the automobile market in North America in order to be perceived as the leader in "safety", whereas BMW has traditionally positioned its brand to be perceived as the leader in "performance".

Ideally, a firm's positioning can be maintained over a long period of time because the company possesses, or can develop, some form of sustainable competitive advantage. The positioning should also be sufficiently relevant to the target segment such that it will drive the purchasing behavior of target customers. To sum up,the marketing branch of a company is to deal with the selling and popularity of its products among people and its customers, as the central and eventual goal of a company is customer satisfaction and the return of revenue.

Implementation Planning

The Marketing Metrics Continuum provides a framework for how to categorize metrics from the tactical to strategic.

If the company has obtained an adequate understanding of the customer base and its own competitive position in the industry, marketing managers are able to make their own key strategic decisions and develop a marketing strategy designed to maximize the revenues and profits of the firm. The selected strategy may aim for any of a variety of specific objectives, including optimizing short-term unit margins, revenue growth, market share, long-term profitability, or other goals.

After the firm's strategic objectives have been identified, the target market selected, and the desired positioning for the company, product or brand has been determined, marketing managers focus on how to best implement the chosen strategy. Traditionally, this has involved implementation planning across the "4 Ps": product management, pricing (at what price slot does a producer position a product, e.g. low, medium or high price), place (the place or area where the products are going to be sold, which could be local, regional, countrywide or international) (i.e. sales and distribution channels), and promotion.

Taken together, the company's implementation choices across the 4 P's are often described as the marketing mix, meaning the mix of elements the business will employ to "go to market" and execute the marketing strategy. The overall goal for the marketing mix is to consistently deliver a compelling value proposition that reinforces the firm's chosen positioning, builds customer loyalty and brand equity among target customers, and achieves the firm's marketing and financial objectives.

In many cases, marketing management will develop a marketing plan to specify how the company will execute the chosen strategy and achieve the business' objectives. The content of marketing plans varies for each firm, but commonly includes:

- An executive summary
- Situation analysis to summarize facts and insights gained from market research and marketing analysis
- The company's mission statement or long-term strategic vision
- A statement of the company's key objectives, often subdivided into marketing objectives and financial objectives
- The marketing strategy the business has chosen, specifying the target segments to be pursued and the competitive positioning to be achieved
- Implementation choices for each element of the marketing mix (the 4 P's)

PROJECT, PROCESS, AND VENDOR MANAGEMENT

More broadly, marketing managers work to design and improve the effectiveness of core marketing processes, such as new product development, brand management, marketing communications, and pricing. Marketers may employ the tools of business process reengineering to ensure these processes are properly designed, and use a variety of process management techniques to keep them operating smoothly.

Effective execution may require management of both internal resources and a variety of external vendors and service providers, such as the firm's advertising agency. Marketers may therefore coordinate with the company's Purchasing department on the procurement of these services. Under the area of marketing agency management (i.e. working with external marketing agencies and suppliers) are techniques such as agency performance evaluation, scope of work, incentive compensation, RFx's and storage of agency information in a supplier database.

Reporting, Measurement, Feedback and Aontrol Systems

Marketing management employs a variety of metrics to measure progress against objectives. It is the responsibility of marketing managers to ensure that the execution of marketing programs achieves the desired objectives and does so in a cost-efficient manner.

Marketing management therefore often makes use of various organizational control systems, such as sales forecasts, and sales force and reseller incentive programs, sales force management systems, and customer relationship management tools (CRM). Some software vendors have begun using the term marketing operations management or marketing resource management to describe systems that facilitate an integrated approach for controlling marketing resources. In some cases, these efforts may be linked to various supply chain management systems, such as enterprise resource planning (ERP), material requirements planning (MRP), efficient consumer response (ECR), and inventory managementsystems.

International Marketing Management

Globalization has led some firms to market beyond the borders of their home countries, making international marketing a part of those firms' marketing strategy. Marketing managers are often responsible for influencing the level, timing, and composition of customer demand. In part, this is because the role of a marketing manager (or sometimes called managing marketer in small- and medium-sized enterprises) can vary significantly based on a business's size, corporate culture, and industry context. For example, in a small- and medium-sized enterprises, the managing marketer may contribute in both managerial and marketing operations roles for the company brands. In a large consumer products company, the marketing manager may act as the overall general manager of his or her assigned product. To create an effective, cost-efficient marketing management strategy, firms must possess a detailed, objective understanding of their own business and the market in which they operate. In analyzing these issues, the discipline of marketing management often overlaps with the related discipline of strategic planning.

2

History of Pharmaceutical Market

The pharmaceutical industry discovers, develops, produces, and markets drugs or pharmaceutical drugs for use as medications to be administered to patients (or self-administered), with the aim to cure them, vaccinate them, or alleviate symptoms. Pharmaceutical companies may deal in generic or brand medications and medical devices. They are subject to a variety of laws and regulations that govern the patenting, testing, safety, efficacy using drug testing and marketing of drugs. The global pharmaceuticals market produced treatments worth $1,228.45 billion in 2020 and showed a compound annual growth rate (CAGR) of 1.8%.

The history of pharmacy as an independent science dates back to the first third of the 19th century. Before then, pharmacy evolved from antiquity as part of medicine. The history of pharmacy coincides well with the history of medicine, but it's important that there is a distinction between the two topics. Pharmaceuticals is one of the most-researched fields in the academic industry, but the history surrounding that particular topic is sparse compared to the impact its made world-wide. Before the advent of pharmacists, there existed apothecaries that worked alongside priests and physicians in regard to patient care.

Notwithstanding, the intensive research work done in different pharmaceutical research fronts such as disposal and fate, environmental impacts and concerns, human health risks, removal, degradation and development of treatment technologies, found that such research is not totally aligned with the market trends and consumption patterns. There are other drivers and interests that promote the pharmaceutical research. Thus, this review is an important contribution to those that are interested not only on the pharmaceutical market and drugs consumption, but also on the links, the drivers and interests that motivate and determine the research work on certain groups of pharmaceuticals on water and wastewater.

Emerging Markets: Self-Pay for Pharmaceuticals

Pharmaceutical markets in developing countries differ from those of industrialized countries in that insurance coverage for drugs is very limited, with most people paying directly out-of-pocket, especially those at lower income levels. Theory suggests that manufacturers might seek to practice price discrimination – charging lower prices in these countries than in higher-income countries – if they were assured that the drugs would not be exported to, or their lower prices would not be referenced by, higher-income countries. Similarly, price discrimination between rich and poor consumers within these countries would also increase sales for companies and access for consumers, if it were feasible. However, government policies, distribution systems, and other factors undermine market segmentation in developing countries, although corporate strategies such as dual branding, direct distribution to providers, and consumer coupons can be effective for some drugs. Inefficient distribution systems also pay a role in raising retail prices to consumers, regardless of prices charged by manufacturers in many developing countries.

The global nature of pharmaceutical R&D raises issues of appropriate cross-national price differentials to share the joint costs. Theoretical models of monopoly pricing using either price discrimination or uniform pricing and models of Ramsey pricing applied to payment for the joint costs of R&D suggest that differential pricing is welfare superior to uniform pricing across countries. Assuming that higher-income countries have more inelastic demand, this implies that richer countries should pay higher prices than poorer countries, and this is consistent with most norms of equity. The principle of differential pricing between the richest and poorest nations is widely accepted in policy debates. However, in practice, consensus breaks down on appropriate price differentials and absolute price levels, particularly for middle-income countries with emerging middle classes but large poor populations.

The evidence suggests that drug prices are higher, relative to average per capita income, in low- and middle-income countries. This applies to generics as well as on-patent drugs. Relatively high prices in low- and middle-income countries partly reflects the highly skewed income distributions, which create incentives for firms to target the more affluent segment (Flynn et al., 2006). Further, because regulatory systems in these countries do not require that generic copies be bioequivalent to the originator, quality uncertainty leads producers to compete on brand, using both brand and high price as a proxy for quality (Danzon et al., 2011). In such markets, only the lowest-quality firms compete on price. However, regulatory requirements for bioequivalence of all generics would likely put many local firms out of business. Thus, the obstacles to reform are primarily political.

HISTORY

Mid-1800s – 1945: From botanicals to the first synthetic drugs

The modern pharmaceutical industry traces its roots to two sources. The first of these were local apothecaries that expanded from their traditional role distributing botanical drugs such as morphine and quinine to wholesale manufacture in the mid 1800s. Rational drug discovery from plants started particularly with the isolation of morphine, analgesic and sleep-inducing agent from opium, by the German apothecary assistant Friedrich Sertürner who named the compound after the Greek god of dreams, Morpheus. By the late 1880s, German dye manufacturers had perfected the purification of individual organic compounds from tar and other mineral sources and had also established rudimentary methods in organic chemical synthesis. The development of synthetic chemical methods allowed scientists to systematically vary the structure of chemical substances, and growth in the emerging science of pharmacology expanded their ability to evaluate the biological effects of these structural changes.

Epinephrine, Norepinephrine, and Amphetamine

By the 1890s, the profound effect of adrenal extracts on many different tissue types had been discovered, setting off a search both for the mechanism of chemical signalling and efforts to exploit these observations for the development of new drugs. The blood pressure raising and vasoconstrictive effects of adrenal extracts were of particular interest to surgeons as hemostatic agents and as treatment for shock, and a number of companies developed products based on adrenal extracts containing varying purities of the active substance. In 1897, John Abel of Johns Hopkins University identified the active principle as epinephrine, which he isolated in an impure state as the sulfate salt. Industrial chemist Jokichi Takamine later developed a method for obtaining epinephrine in a pure state, and licensed the technology to Parke-Davis. Parke-Davis marketed epinephrine under the trade name Adrenalin. Injected epinephrine proved to be especially efficacious for the acute treatment of asthma attacks, and an inhaled version was sold in the United States until 2011 (Primatene Mist). By 1929 epinephrine had been formulated into an inhaler for use in the treatment of nasal congestion.

While highly effective, the requirement for injection limited the use of epinephrine and orally active derivatives were sought. A structurally similar compound, ephedrine, (actually more similar to norepinephrine,) was identified by Japanese chemists in the Ma Huang plant and marketed by Eli Lilly as an oral treatment for asthma. Following the work of Henry Dale and George Barger at Burroughs-Wellcome, academic chemist Gordon Alles synthesized amphetamine and tested it in asthma patients in 1929. The drug proved to have only modest anti-asthma effects, but produced sensations of exhilaration and palpitations. Amphetamine was developed by Smith, Kline and French as a nasal decongestant under the trade name Benzedrine Inhaler. Amphetamine was eventually developed for the treatment of narcolepsy, post-encephalitic parkinsonism, and mood elevation in depression and other psychiatric indications. It received approval as a New and Nonofficial Remedy from the American Medical Association for these uses in 1937 and remained in common use for depression until the development of tricyclic antidepressants in the 1960s.

Discovery and Development of the Barbiturates

In 1903, Hermann Emil Fischer and Joseph von Mering disclosed their discovery that diethylbarbituric acid, formed from the reaction of diethylmalonic acid, phosphorus oxychloride and urea, induces sleep in dogs. The discovery was patented and licensed to Bayer pharmaceuticals, which marketed the compound under the trade name Veronal as a sleep aid beginning in 1904. Systematic investigations of the effect of structural changes on potency and duration of action led to the discovery of phenobarbital at Bayer in 1911 and the discovery of its potent anti-epileptic activity in 1912. Phenobarbital was among the most widely used drugs for the treatment of epilepsy through the 1970s, and as of 2014, remains on the World Health Organizations list of essential medications. The 1950s and 1960s saw increased awareness of the addictive properties and abuse potential of barbiturates and amphetamines and led to increasing restrictions on their use and growing government oversight of prescribers. Today, amphetamine is largely restricted to use in the treatment of attention deficit disorder and phenobarbital in the treatment of epilepsy.

Insulin

A series of experiments performed from the late 1800s to the early 1900s revealed that diabetes is caused by the absence of a substance normally produced by the pancreas. In 1869, Oskar Minkowski and Joseph von Mering found that diabetes could be induced in dogs by surgical removal of the pancreas. In 1921, Canadian professor Frederick Banting and his student Charles Best repeated this study, and found that injections of pancreatic extract reversed the symptoms produced by pancreas removal. Soon, the extract was demonstrated to work in people, but development of insulin therapy as a routine medical procedure was delayed by difficulties in producing the material in sufficient quantity and with reproducible purity. The researchers sought assistance from industrial collaborators at Eli Lilly and Co. based on the company's experience with large scale purification of biological materials. Chemist George B. Walden of Eli Lilly and Company found that careful adjustment of the pH of the extract allowed a relatively pure grade of insulin to be produced. Under pressure from Toronto University and a potential patent challenge by academic scientists who had independently developed a similar purification method, an agreement was reached for non-exclusive production of insulin by multiple companies. Prior to the discovery and widespread availability of insulin therapy the life expectancy of diabetics was only a few months.

Early anti-infective research: Salvarsan, Prontosil, Penicillin and vaccines

The development of drugs for the treatment of infectious diseases was a major focus of early research and development efforts; in 1900 pneumonia, tuberculosis, and diarrhea were the three leading causes of death in the United States and mortality in the first year of life exceeded 10%.

In 1911 arsphenamine, the first synthetic anti-infective drug, was developed by Paul Ehrlich and chemist Alfred Bertheim of the Institute of Experimental Therapy in Berlin. The drug was given the commercial name Salvarsan. Ehrlich, noting both the general toxicity of arsenic and the selective absorption of certain dyes by bacteria, hypothesized that an arsenic-containing dye with similar selective absorption properties could be used to treat bacterial infections. Arsphenamine was prepared as part of a campaign to synthesize a series of such compounds, and found to exhibit partially selective toxicity. Arsphenamine proved to be the first effective treatment for syphilis, a disease which prior to that time was incurable and led inexorably to severe skin ulceration, neurological damage, and death.

Ehrlich's approach of systematically varying the chemical structure of synthetic compounds and measuring the effects of these changes on biological activity was pursued broadly by industrial scientists, including Bayer scientists Josef Klarer, Fritz Mietzsch, and Gerhard Domagk. This work, also based in the testing of compounds available from the German dye industry, led to the development of Prontosil, the first representative of the sulfonamide class of antibiotics. Compared to arsphenamine, the sulfonamides had a broader spectrum of activity and were far less toxic, rendering them useful for infections caused by pathogens such as streptococci. In 1939, Domagk received the Nobel Prize in Medicine for this discovery. Nonetheless, the dramatic decrease in deaths from infectious diseases that occurred prior to World War II was primarily the result of improved public health measures such as clean water and less crowded housing, and the impact of anti-infective drugs and vaccines was significant mainly after World War II.

In 1928, Alexander Fleming discovered the antibacterial effects of penicillin, but its exploitation for the treatment of human disease awaited the development of methods for its large scale production and purification. These were developed by a U.S. and British government-led consortium of pharmaceutical companies during the Second World War.

Early progress toward the development of vaccines occurred throughout this period, primarily in the form of academic and government-funded basic research directed toward the identification of the pathogens responsible for common communicable diseases. In 1885 Louis Pasteur and Pierre Paul Émile Roux created the first rabies vaccine. The first diphtheria vaccines were produced in 1914 from a mixture of diphtheria toxin and antitoxin (produced from the serum of an inoculated animal), but the safety of the inoculation was marginal and it was not widely used. The United States recorded 206,000 cases of diphtheria in 1921 resulting in 15,520 deaths. In 1923 parallel efforts by Gaston Ramon at the Pasteur Institute and Alexander Glenny at the Wellcome Research Laboratories (later part of GlaxoSmithKline) led to the discovery that a safer vaccine could be produced by treating diphtheria toxin with formaldehyde. In 1944, Maurice Hilleman of Squibb Pharmaceuticals developed the first vaccine against Japanese encephelitis. Hilleman would later move to Merck where he would play a key role in the development of vaccines against measles, mumps, chickenpox, rubella, hepatitis A, hepatitis B, and meningitis.

Unsafe Drugs and Early Industry Regulation

Prior to the 20th century drugs were generally produced by small scale manufacturers with little regulatory control over manufacturing or claims of safety and efficacy. To the extent that such laws did exist, enforcement was lax. In the United States, increased regulation of vaccines and other biological drugs was spurred by tetanus outbreaks and deaths caused by the distribution of contaminated smallpox vaccine and diphtheria antitoxin. The Biologics Control Act of 1902 required that federal government grant premarket approval for every biological drug and for the process and facility producing such drugs. This was followed in 1906 by the Pure Food and Drugs Act, which forbade the interstate distribution of adulterated or misbranded foods and drugs. A drug was considered misbranded if it contained alcohol, morphine, opium, cocaine, or any of several other potentially dangerous or addictive drugs, and if its label failed to indicate the quantity or proportion of such drugs. The government's attempts to use the law to prosecute manufacturers for making unsupported claims of efficacy were undercut by a Supreme Court ruling restricting the federal government's enforcement powers to cases of incorrect specification of the drug's ingredients.

In 1937 over 100 people died after ingesting "Elixir Sulfanilamide" manufactured by S.E. Massengill Company of Tennessee. The product was formulated in diethylene glycol, a highly toxic solvent that is now widely used as antifreeze. Under the laws extant at that time, prosecution of the manufacturer was possible only under the technicality that the product had been called an "elixir", which literally implied a solution in ethanol. In response to this episode, the U.S. Congress passed the Federal Food, Drug, and Cosmetic Act of 1938, which for the first time required pre-market demonstration of safety before a drug could be sold, and explicitly prohibited false therapeutic claims.

The Post-War Years, 1945–1970

Further advances in anti-infective research

The aftermath of World War II saw an explosion in the discovery of new classes of antibacterial drugs including the cephalosporins (developed by Eli Lilly based on the seminal work of Giuseppe Brotzu and Edward Abraham), streptomycin (discovered during a Merck-funded research program in Selman Waksman's laboratory), the tetracyclines(discovered at Lederle Laboratories, now a part of Pfizer), erythromycin (discovered at Eli Lilly and Co.) and their extension to an increasingly wide range of bacterial pathogens. Streptomycin, discovered during a Merck-funded research program in Selman Waksman's laboratory at Rutgers in 1943, became the first effective treatment for tuberculosis. At the time of its discovery, sanitoriums for the isolation of tuberculosis-infected people were an ubiquitous feature of cities in developed countries, with 50% dying within 5 years of admission.

A Federal Trade Commission report issued in 1958 attempted to quantify the effect of antibiotic development on American public health. The report found that over the period 1946-1955, there was a 42% drop in the incidence of diseases for which antibiotics were effective and only a 20% drop in those for which antibiotics were not effective. The report concluded that "it appears that the use of antibiotics, early diagnosis, and other factors have limited the epidemic spread and thus the number of these diseases which have occurred". The study further examined mortality rates for eight common diseases for which antibiotics offered effective therapy (syphilis, tuberculosis, dysentery, scarlet fever, whooping cough, meningococcal infections, and pneumonia), and found a 56% decline over the same period. Notable among these was a 75% decline in deaths due to tuberculosis.

During the years 1940-1955, the rate of decline in the U.S. death rate accelerated from 2% per year to 8% per year, then returned to the historical rate of 2% per year. The dramatic decline in the immediate post-war years has been attributed to the rapid development of new treatments and vaccines for infectious disease that occurred during these years. Vaccine development continued to accelerate, with the most notable achievement of the period being Jonas Salk's 1954 development of the polio vaccine under the funding of the non-profit National Foundation for Infantile Paralysis. The vaccine process was never patented, but was instead given to pharmaceutical companies to manufacture as a low-cost generic. In 1960 Maurice Hilleman of Merck Sharp & Dohme identified the SV40 virus, which was later shown to cause tumors in many mammalian species. It was later determined that SV40 was present as a contaminant in polio vaccine lots that had been administered to 90% of the children in the United States. The contamination appears to have originated both in the original cell stock and in monkey tissue used for production. In 2004 the United States Cancer Institute announced that it had concluded that SV40 is not associated with cancer in people.

Other notable new vaccines of the period include those for measles (1962, John Franklin Enders of Children's Medical Center Boston, later refined by Maurice Hilleman at Merck), Rubella (1969, Hilleman, Merck) and mumps (1967, Hilleman, Merck) The United States incidences of rubella, congenital rubella syndrome, measles, and mumps all fell by >95% in the immediate aftermath of widespread vaccination. The first 20 years of licensed measles vaccination in the U.S. prevented an estimated 52 million cases of the disease, 17,400 cases of mental retardation, and 5,200 deaths.

Development and Marketing of Antihypertensive Drugs

Hypertension is a risk factor for atherosclerosis, heart failure, coronary artery disease, stroke, renal disease, and peripheral arterial disease, and is the most important risk factor for cardiovascular morbidity and mortality, in industrialized countries. Prior to 1940 approximately 23% of all deaths among persons over age 50 were attributed to hypertension. Severe cases of hypertension were treated by surgery.

Early developments in the field of treating hypertension included quaternary ammonium ion sympathetic nervous system blocking agents, but these compounds were never widely used due to their severe side effects, because the long term health consequences of high blood pressure had not yet been established, and because they had to be administered by injection.

In 1952 researchers at Ciba discovered the first orally available vasodilator, hydralazine. A major shortcoming of hydralazine monotherapy was that it lost its effectiveness over time (tachyphylaxis). In the mid-1950s Karl H. Beyer, James M. Sprague, John E. Baer, and Frederick C. Novello of Merck and Co. discovered and developed chlorothiazide, which remains the most widely used antihypertensive drug today. This development was associated with a substantial decline in the mortality rate among people with hypertension.The inventors were recognized by a Public Health Lasker Award in 1975 for "the saving of untold thousands of lives and the alleviation of the suffering of millions of victims of hypertension".

A 2009 Cochrane review concluded that thiazide antihypertensive drugs reduce the risk of death (RR 0.89), stroke (RR 0.63), coronary heart disease (RR 0.84), and cardiovascular events (RR 0.70) in people with high blood pressure. In the ensuring years other classes of antihypertensive drug were developed and found wide acceptance in combination therapy, including loop diuretics (Lasix/furosemide, Hoechst Pharmaceuticals, 1963), beta blockers (ICI Pharmaceuticals, 1964) ACE inhibitors, and angiotensin receptor blockers. ACE inhibitors reduce the risk of new onset kidney disease [RR 0.71] and death [RR 0.84] in diabetic patients, irrespective of whether they have hypertension.

Oral Contraceptives

Prior to the second world war, birth control was prohibited in many countries, and in the United States even the discussion of contraceptive methods sometimes led to prosecution under Comstock laws. The history of the development of oral contraceptives is thus closely tied to the birth control movement and the efforts of activists Margaret Sanger, Mary Dennett, and Emma Goldman. Based on fundamental research performed by Gregory Pincus and synthetic methods for progesterone developed by Carl Djerassi at Syntex and by Frank Colton at G.D. Searle & Co., the first oral contraceptive, Enovid, was developed by E.D. Searle and Co. and approved by the FDA in 1960. The original formulation incorporated vastly excessive doses of hormones, and caused severe side effects. Nonetheless, by 1962, 1.2 million American women were on the pill, and by 1965 the number had increased to 6.5 million. The availability of a convenient form of temporary contraceptive led to dramatic changes in social mores including expanding the range of lifestyle options available to women, reducing the reliance of women on men for contraceptive practice, encouraging the delay of marriage, and increasing pre-marital co-habitation.

Thalidomide and the Kefauver-Harris Amendments

In the U.S., a push for revisions of the FD&C Act emerged from Congressional hearings led by Senator Estes Kefauver of Tennessee in 1959. The hearings covered a wide range of policy issues, including advertising abuses, questionable efficacy of drugs, and the need for greater regulation of the industry. While momentum for new legislation temporarily flagged under extended debate, a new tragedy emerged that underscored the need for more comprehensive regulation and provided the driving force for the passage of new laws.

On 12 September 1960, an American licensee, the William S. Merrell Company of Cincinnati, submitted a new drug application for Kevadon (thalidomide), a sedative that had been marketed in Europe since 1956. The FDA medical officer in charge of reviewing the compound, Frances Kelsey, believed that the data supporting the safety of thalidomide was incomplete. The firm continued to pressure Kelsey and the FDA to approve the application until November 1961, when the drug was pulled off the German market because of its association with grave congenital abnormalities. Several thousand newborns in Europe and elsewhere suffered the teratogenic effects of thalidomide. Without approval from the FDA, the firm distributed Kevadon to over 1,000 physicians there under the guise of investigational use. Over 20,000 Americans received thalidomide in this "study," including 624 pregnant patients, and about 17 known newborns suffered the effects of the drug.

The thalidomide tragedy resurrected Kefauver's bill to enhance drug regulation that had stalled in Congress, and the Kefauver-Harris Amendment became law on 10 October 1962. Manufacturers henceforth had to prove to FDA that their drugs were effective as well as safe before they could go on the US market. The FDA received authority to regulate advertising of prescription drugs and to establish good manufacturing practices. The law required that all drugs introduced between 1938 and 1962 had to be effective. An FDA - National Academy of Sciences collaborative study showed that nearly 40 percent of these products were not effective. A similarly comprehensive study of over-the-counter products began ten years later.

1970–1980s

Statins

In 1971, Akira Endo, a Japanese biochemist working for the pharmaceutical company Sankyo, identified mevastatin (ML-236B), a molecule produced by the fungus Penicillium citrinum, as an inhibitor of HMG-CoA reductase, a critical enzyme used by the body to produce cholesterol. Animal trials showed very good inhibitory effect as in clinical trials, however a long term study in dogs found toxic effects at higher doses and as a result mevastatin was believed to be too toxic for human use. Mevastatin was never marketed, because of its adverse effects of tumors, muscle deterioration, and sometimes death in laboratory dogs.

P. Roy Vagelos, chief scientist and later CEO of Merck & Co, was interested, and made several trips to Japan starting in 1975. By 1978, Merck had isolated lovastatin (mevinolin, MK803) from the fungus Aspergillus terreus, first marketed in 1987 as Mevacor.

In April 1994, the results of a Merck-sponsored study, the Scandinavian Simvastatin Survival Study, were announced. Researchers tested simvastatin, later sold by Merck as Zocor, on 4,444 patients with high cholesterol and heart disease. After five years, the study concluded the patients saw a 35% reduction in their cholesterol, and their chances of dying of a heart attack were reduced by 42%. In 1995, Zocor and Mevacor both made Merck over US$1 billion. Endo was awarded the 2006 Japan Prize, and the Lasker-DeBakey Clinical Medical Research Award in 2008. For his "pioneering research into a new class of molecules" for "lowering cholesterol,"

Research and development

Drug discovery is the process by which potential drugs are discovered or designed. In the past most drugs have been discovered either by isolating the active ingredient from traditional remedies or by serendipitous discovery. Modern biotechnology often focuses on understanding the metabolic pathways related to a disease state or pathogen, and manipulating these pathways using molecular biology or biochemistry. A great deal of early-stage drug discovery has traditionally been carried out by universities and research institutions.

Drug development refers to activities undertaken after a compound is identified as a potential drug in order to establish its suitability as a medication. Objectives of drug development are to determine appropriate formulation and dosing, as well as to establish safety. Research in these areas generally includes a combination of in vitro studies, in vivostudies, and clinical trials. The cost of late stage development has meant it is usually done by the larger pharmaceutical companies.

Often, large multinational corporations exhibit vertical integration, participating in a broad range of drug discovery and development, manufacturing and quality control, marketing, sales, and distribution. Smaller organizations, on the other hand, often focus on a specific aspect such as discovering drug candidates or developing formulations. Often, collaborative agreements between research organizations and large pharmaceutical companies are formed to explore the potential of new drug substances. More recently, multi-nationals are increasingly relying on contract research organizations to manage drug development.

The cost of Innovation

Drug discovery and development is very expensive; of all compounds investigated for use in humans only a small fraction are eventually approved in most nations by government appointed medical institutions or boards, who have to approve new drugs before they can be marketed in those countries. In 2010 18 NMEs (New Molecular Entities) were approved and three biologics by the FDA, or 21 in total, which is down from 26 in 2009 and 24 in 2008. On the other hand, there were only 18 approvals in total in 2007 and 22 back in 2006. Since 2001, the Center for Drug Evaluation and Research has averaged 22.9 approvals a year. This approval comes only after heavy investment in pre-clinical development and clinical trials, as well as a commitment to ongoing safety monitoring. Drugs which fail part-way through this process often incur large costs, while generating no revenue in return. If the cost of these failed drugs is taken into account, the cost of developing a successful new drug (new chemical entity, or NCE), has been estimated at about US$1.3 billion(not including marketing expenses). Professors Light and Lexchin reported in 2012, however, that the rate of approval for new drugs has been a relatively stable average rate of 15 to 25 for decades.

Industry-wide research and investment reached a record $65.3 billion in 2009. While the cost of research in the U.S. was about $34.2 billion between 1995 and 2010, revenues rose faster (revenues rose by $200.4 billion in that time).

A study by the consulting firm Bain & Company reported that the cost for discovering, developing and launching (which factored in marketing and other business expenses) a new drug (along with the prospective drugs that fail) rose over a five-year period to nearly $1.7 billion in 2003. According to Forbes, by 2010 development costs were between $4 billion to $11 billion per drug.

Some of these estimates also take into account the opportunity cost of investing capital many years before revenues are realized (see Time-value of money). Because of the very long time needed for discovery, development, and approval of pharmaceuticals, these costs can accumulate to nearly half the total expense. A direct consequence within the pharmaceutical industry value chain is that major pharmaceutical multinationals tend to increasingly outsource risks related to fundamental research, which somewhat reshapes the industry ecosystem with biotechnology companies playing an increasingly important role, and overall strategies being redefined accordingly. Some approved drugs, such as those based on re-formulation of an existing active ingredient (also referred to as Line-extensions) are much less expensive to develop.

Controversies

Due to repeated accusations and findings that some clinical trials conducted or funded by pharmaceutical companies may report only positive results for the preferred medication, the industry has been looked at much more closely by independent groups and government agencies.

In response to specific cases in which unfavorable data from pharmaceutical company-sponsored research was not published, the Pharmaceutical Research and Manufacturers of America have published new guidelines urging companies to report all findings and limit the financial involvement in drug companies of researchers. US congress signed into law a bill which requires phase II and phase III clinical trials to be registered by the sponsor on the clinicaltrials.gov website run by the NIH.

Drug researchers not directly employed by pharmaceutical companies often look to companies for grants, and companies often look to researchers for studies that will make their products look favorable. Sponsored researchers are rewarded by drug companies, for example with support for their conference/symposium costs. Lecture scripts and even journal articles presented by academic researchers may actually be "ghost-written" by pharmaceutical companies.

An investigation by ProPublica found that at least 21 doctors have been paid more than $500,000 for speeches and consulting by drugs manufacturers since 2009, with half of the top earners working in psychiatry, and about $2 billion in total paid to doctors for such services. AstraZeneca, Johnson & Johnson and Eli Lilly have paid billions of dollars in federal settlements over allegations that they paid doctors to promote drugs for unapproved uses. Some prominent medical schools have since tightened rules on faculty acceptance of such payments by drug companies.

In contrast to this viewpoint, an article and associated editorial in the New England Journal of Medicine in May 2015 emphasized the importance of pharmaceutical industry-physician interactions for the development of novel treatments, and argued that moral outrage over industry malfeasance had unjustifiably led many to overemphasize the problems created by financial conflicts of interest. The article noted that major healthcare organizations such as National Center for Advancing Translational Sciences of the National Institutes of Health, the President's Council of Advisors on Science and Technology, the World Economic Forum, the Gates Foundation, the Wellcome Trust, and the Food and Drug Administration had encouraged greater interactions between physicians and industry in order to bring greater benefits to patients.

Product Approval

In the United States, new pharmaceutical products must be approved by the Food and Drug Administration (FDA) as being both safe and effective. This process generally involves submission of an Investigational New Drug filing with sufficient pre-clinical data to support proceeding with human trials. Following IND approval, three phases of progressively larger human clinical trials may be conducted. Phase I generally studies toxicity using healthy volunteers. Phase II can include pharmacokinetics and dosing in patients, and Phase III is a very large study of efficacy in the intended patient population. Following the successful completion of phase III testing, a New Drug Application is submitted to the FDA. The FDA review the data and if the product is seen as having a positive benefit-risk assessment, approval to market the product in the US is granted.

A fourth phase of post-approval surveillance is also often required due to the fact that even the largest clinical trials cannot effectively predict the prevalence of rare side-effects. Postmarketing surveillance ensures that after marketing the safety of a drug is monitored closely. In certain instances, its indication may need to be limited to particular patient groups, and in others the substance is withdrawn from the market completely.

The FDA provides information about approved drugs at the Orange Book site.

In the UK, the Medicines and Healthcare Products Regulatory Agency approves drugs for use, though the evaluation is done by the European Medicines Agency, an agency of the European Union based in London. Normally an approval in the UK and other European countries comes later than one in the USA. Then it is the National Institute for Health and Care Excellence (NICE), for England and Wales, who decides if and how the National Health Service (NHS) will allow (in the sense of paying for) their use. The British National Formulary is the core guide for pharmacists and clinicians.

In many non-US western countries a 'fourth hurdle' of cost effectiveness analysis has developed before new technologies can be provided. This focuses on the efficiency (in terms of the cost per QALY) of the technologies in question rather than their efficacy. In England and Wales NICE decides whether and in what circumstances drugs and technologies will be made available by the NHS, whilst similar arrangements exist with the Scottish Medicines Consortium in Scotland, and the Pharmaceutical Benefits Advisory Committee in Australia. A product must pass the threshold for cost-effectiveness if it is to be approved. Treatments must represent 'value for money' and a net benefit to society.

Orphan drugs

There are special rules for certain rare diseases ("orphan diseases") in several major drug regulatory territories. For example, diseases involving fewer than 200,000 patients in the United States, or larger populations in certain circumstances are subject to the Orphan Drug Act. Because medical research and development of drugs to treat such diseases is financially disadvantageous, companies that do so are rewarded with tax reductions, fee waivers, and market exclusivity on that drug for a limited time (seven years), regardless of whether the drug is protected by patents.

Global sales

In 2011, global spending on prescription drugs topped $954 billion, even as growth slowed somewhat in Europe and North America. The United States accounts for more than a third of the global pharmaceutical market, with $340 billion in annual sales followed by the EU and Japan. Emerging markets such as China, Russia, South Korea and Mexico outpaced that market, growing a huge 81 percent.

The top ten best-selling drugs of 2013 totaled $75.6 billion in sales, with the anti-inflammatory drug Humira being the best-selling drug worldwide at $10.7 billion in sales. The second and third best selling were Enbrel and Remicade, respectively. The top three best-selling drugs in the United States in 2013 were Abilify ($6.3 billion,) Nexium ($6 billion) and Humira ($5.4 billion). The best-selling drug ever, Lipitor, averaged $13 billion annually and netted $141 billion total over its lifetime before Pfizer's patent expired in November 2011.

IMS Health publishes an analysis of trends expected in the pharmaceutical industry in 2007, including increasing profits in most sectors despite loss of some patents, and new 'blockbuster' drugs on the horizon.

Patents and Generics

Depending on a number of considerations, a company may apply for and be granted a patent for the drug, or the process of producing the drug, granting exclusivity rights typically for about 20 years. However, only after rigorous study and testing, which takes 10 to 15 years on average, will governmental authorities grant permission for the company to market and sell the drug. Patent protection enables the owner of the patent to recover the costs of research and development through high profit margins for the branded drug. When the patent protection for the drug expires, a generic drug is usually developed and sold by a competing company. The development and approval of generics is less expensive, allowing them to be sold at a lower price. Often the owner of the branded drug will introduce a generic version before the patent expires in order to get a head start in the generic market.Restructuring has therefore become routine, driven by the patent expiration of products launched during the industry's "golden era" in the 1990s and companies' failure to develop sufficient new blockbuster products to replace lost revenues.

Prescriptions

In the U.S., the value of prescriptions increased over the period of 1995 to 2005 by 3.4 billion annually, a 61 percent increase. Retail sales of prescription drugs jumped 250 percent from $72 billion to $250 billion, while the average price of prescriptions more than doubled from $30 to $68.

Marketing

Advertising is common in healthcare journals as well as through more mainstream media routes. In some countries, notably the US, they are allowed to advertise directly to the general public. Pharmaceutical companies generally employ sales people (often called 'drug reps' or, an older term, 'detail men') to market directly and personally to physicians and other healthcare providers. In some countries, notably the US, pharmaceutical companies also employ lobbyists to influence politicians. Marketing of prescription drugs in the US is regulated by the federal Prescription Drug Marketing Act of 1987.

To Healthcare Professionals

The book Bad Pharma also discusses the influence of drug representatives, how ghostwriters are employed by the drug companies to write papers for academics to publish, how independent the academic journals really are, how the drug companies finance doctors' continuing education, and how patients' groups are often funded by industry.

Direct to Consumer Advertising

Since the 1980s new methods of marketing for prescription drugs to consumers have become important. Direct-to-consumer media advertising was legalised in the FDA Guidance for Industry on Consumer-Directed Broadcast Advertisements.

CONTROVERSY ABOUT DRUG MARKETING AND LOBBYING

There has been increasing controversy surrounding pharmaceutical marketing and influence. There have been accusations and findings of influence on doctors and other health professionals through drug reps including the constant provision of marketing 'gifts' and biased information to health professionals; highly prevalent advertising in journals and conferences; funding independent healthcare organizations and health promotion campaigns; lobbying physicians and politicians (more than any other industry in the US); sponsorship of medical schools or nurse training; sponsorship of continuing educational events, with influence on the curriculum; and hiring physicians as paid consultants on medical advisory boards.

Some advocacy groups, such as No Free Lunch and AllTrials, have criticized the effect of drug marketing to physicians because they say it biases physicians to prescribe the marketed drugs even when others might be cheaper or better for the patient.

There have been related accusations of disease mongering(over-medicalising) to expand the market for medications. An inaugural conference on that subject took place in Australia in 2006. In 2009, the Government-funded National Prescribing Service launched the "Finding Evidence – Recognising Hype" program, aimed at educating GPs on methods for independent drug analysis.

A 2005 review by a special committee of the UK government came to all the above conclusions in a European Union context whilst also highlighting the contributions and needs of the industry.

Meta-analyses have shown that psychiatric studies sponsored by pharmaceutical companies are several times more likely to report positive results, and if a drug company employee is involved the effect is even larger. Influence has also extended to the training of doctors and nurses in medical schools, which is being fought.

It has been argued that the design of the Diagnostic and Statistical Manual of Mental Disorders and the expansion of the criteria represents an increasing medicalization of human nature, or "disease mongering", driven by drug company influence on psychiatry. The potential for direct conflict of interest has been raised, partly because roughly half the authors who selected and defined the DSM-IV psychiatric disorders had or previously had financial relationships with the pharmaceutical industry.

In the US, starting in 2013, under the Physician Financial Transparency Reports (part of the Sunshine Act), the Centers for Medicare & Medicaid Services has to collect information from applicable manufacturers and group purchasing organizations in order to report information about their financial relationships with physicians and hospitals. Data are made public in the Centers for Medicare & Medicaid Services website. The expectation is that relationship between doctors and Pharmaceutical industry will become fully transparent.

In a report conducted by the Center for Responsive Politics, there were more than 1,100 lobbyists working in some capacity for the pharmaceutical business in 2017. In the first quarter of 2017, the health products and pharmaceutical industry spent $78 million on lobbying members of the United States Congress.

Regulatory Issues

Ben Goldacre has argued that regulators – such as the Medicines and Healthcare products Regulatory Agency (MHRA) in the UK, or the Food and Drug Administration (FDA) in the United States – advance the interests of the drug companies rather than the interests of the public due to revolving door exchange of employees between the regulator and the companies and friendships develop between regulator and company employees. He argues that regulators do not require that new drugs offer an improvement over what is already available, or even that they be particularly effective.

Others have argued that excessive regulation suppresses therapeutic innovation, and that the current cost of regulator-required clinical trials prevents the full exploitation of new genetic and biological knowledge for the treatment of human disease. A 2012 report by the President's Council of Advisors on Science and Technology made several key recommendations to reduce regulatory burdens to new drug development, including 1) expanding the FDA's use of accelerated approval processes, 2) creating an expedited approval pathway for drugs intended for use in narrowly defined populations, and 3) undertaking pilot projects designed to evaluate the feasibility of a new, adaptive drug approval process.

PHARMACEUTICAL FRAUD

Pharmaceutical fraud involves deceptions which bring financial gain to a pharmaceutical company. It affects individuals and public and private insurers. There are several different schemes used to defraud the health care system which are particular to the pharmaceutical industry. These include: Good Manufacturing Practice (GMP) Violations, Off Label Marketing, Best Price Fraud, CME Fraud, Medicaid Price Reporting, and Manufactured Compound Drugs. Of this amount $2.5 billion was recovered through False Claims Actcases in FY 2010. Examples of fraud cases include the GlaxoSmithKline $3 billion settlement, Pfizer $2.3 billion settlement and Merck & Co. $650 million settlement. Damages from fraud can be recovered by use of the False Claims Act, most commonly under the qui tam provisions which rewards an individual for being a "whistleblower", or relator (law).

Every major company selling the antipsychotics — Bristol-Myers Squibb, Eli Lilly, Pfizer, AstraZeneca and Johnson & Johnson — has either settled recent government cases, under the False Claims Act, for hundreds of millions of dollars or is currently under investigation for possible health care fraud. Following charges of illegal marketing, two of the settlements set records last year for the largest criminal fines ever imposed on corporations. One involved Eli Lilly's antipsychotic Zyprexa, and the other involved Bextra. In the Bextra case, the government also charged Pfizer with illegally marketing another antipsychotic, Geodon; Pfizer settled that part of the claim for $301 million, without admitting any wrongdoing.

On 2 July 2012, GlaxoSmithKline pleaded guilty to criminal charges and agreed to a $3 billion settlement of the largest health-care fraud case in the U.S. and the largest payment by a drug company. The settlement is related to the company's illegal promotion of prescription drugs, its failure to report safety data, bribing doctors, and promoting medicines for uses for which they were not licensed. The drugs involved were Paxil, Wellbutrin, Advair, Lamictal, and Zofran for off-label, non-covered uses. Those and the drugs Imitrex, Lotronex, Flovent, and Valtrex were involved in the kickback scheme.

The following is a list of the four largest settlements reached with pharmaceutical companies from 1991 to 2012, rank ordered by the size of the total settlement. Legal claims against the pharmaceutical industry have varied widely over the past two decades, including Medicare and Medicaid fraud, off-label promotion, and inadequate manufacturing practices.Pharmaceutical fraud involves deceptions which bring financial gain to a pharmaceutical company. It affects individuals and public and private insurers. There are several different schemes used to defraud the health care system which are particular to the pharmaceutical industry. These include: Good Manufacturing Practice (GMP) Violations, Off Label Marketing, Best Price Fraud, CME Fraud, Medicaid Price Reporting, and Manufactured Compound Drugs. Of this amount $2.5 billion was recovered through False Claims Actcases in FY 2010. Examples of fraud cases include the GlaxoSmithKline $3 billion settlement, Pfizer $2.3 billion settlement and Merck & Co. $650 million settlement. Damages from fraud can be recovered by use of the False Claims Act, most commonly under the qui tam provisions which rewards an individual for being a "whistleblower", or relator (law).

Every major company selling the antipsychotics — Bristol-Myers Squibb, Eli Lilly, Pfizer, AstraZeneca and Johnson & Johnson — has either settled recent government cases, under the False Claims Act, for hundreds of millions of dollars or is currently under investigation for possible health care fraud. Following charges of illegal marketing, two of the settlements set records last year for the largest criminal fines ever imposed on corporations. One involved Eli Lilly's antipsychotic

Zyprexa, and the other involved Bextra. In the Bextra case, the government also charged Pfizer with illegally marketing another antipsychotic, Geodon; Pfizer settled that part of the claim for $301 million, without admitting any wrongdoing.

On 2 July 2012, GlaxoSmithKline pleaded guilty to criminal charges and agreed to a $3 billion settlement of the largest health-care fraud case in the U.S. and the largest payment by a drug company. The settlement is related to the company's illegal promotion of prescription drugs, its failure to report safety data, bribing doctors, and promoting medicines for uses for which they were not licensed. The drugs involved were Paxil, Wellbutrin, Advair, Lamictal, and Zofran for off-label, non-covered uses. Those and the drugs Imitrex, Lotronex, Flovent, and Valtrex were involved in the kickback scheme.

The following is a list of the four largest settlements reached with pharmaceutical companies from 1991 to 2012, rank ordered by the size of the total settlement. Legal claims against the pharmaceutical industry have varied widely over the past two decades, including Medicare and Medicaid fraud, off-label promotion, and inadequate manufacturing practices.

Developing world

Patents

Patents have been criticized in the developing world, as they are thought to reduce access to existing medicines. Reconciling patents and universal access to medicine would require an efficient international policy of price discrimination. Moreover, under the TRIPS agreement of the World Trade Organization, countries must allow pharmaceutical products to be patented. In 2001, the WTO adopted the Doha Declaration, which indicates that the TRIPS agreement should be read with the goals of public health in mind, and allows some methods for circumventing pharmaceutical monopolies: via compulsory licensing or parallel imports, even before patent expiration.

In March 2001, 40 multi-national pharmaceutical companies brought litigation against South Africa for its Medicines Act, which allowed the generic production of antiretroviral drugs (ARVs) for treating HIV, despite the fact that these drugs were on-patent. HIV was and is an epidemic in South Africa, and ARVs at the time cost between 10,000 and US$15,000 per patient per year. This was unaffordable for most South African citizens, and so the South African government committed to providing ARVs at prices closer to what people could afford. To do so, they would need to ignore the patents on drugs and produce generics within the country (using a compulsory license), or import them from abroad. After international protest in favour of public health rights (including the collection of 250,000 signatures by MSF), the governments of several developed countries (including The Netherlands, Germany, France, and later the US) backed the South African government, and the case was dropped in April of that year.

In 2016, GlaxoSmithKline (the worlds 6th largest Pharmaceutical) announced that it would be dropping its patents in poor countries so as to allow independent companies to make and sell versions of its drugs in those areas, thereby widening the public access to them. GlaxoSmithKline published a list of 50 countries they would no longer hold patents in, affecting 1 billion people worldwide.

Charitable Programs

In 2011 four of the top 20 corporate charitable donations and eight of the top 30 corporate charitable donations came from pharmaceutical manufacturers. The bulk of corporate charitable donations (69% as of 2012) comes by way of non-cash charitable donations, the majority of which again were donations contributed by pharmaceutical companies. Some of those large pharmaceutical companies are "patient assistance" foundations, providing financial support to individuals in purchasing prescription medicines, but pharmaceutical companies are also huge givers of in-kind products, i.e. presumably their own drugs. Non-cash donations of product can be "profit maximizing…as part of an inventory control issue when they have excess inventories" for some corporations, says Patrick Rooney of Giving USA in an interview with Nonprofit Quarterly.

Charitable programs and drug discovery & development efforts by pharmaceutical companies include:

- "Merck's Gift", wherein billions of river blindness drugs were donated in Africa
- Pfizer's gift of free/discounted fluconazole and other drugs for AIDS in South Africa
- GSK's commitment to give free albendazole tablets to the WHO for, and until, the elimination of lymphatic filariasis worldwide.
- In 2006, Novartis committed US$755 million in corporate citizenship initiatives around the world, particularly focusing on improving access to medicines in the developing world through its Access to Medicine projects, including donations of medicines to patients affected by leprosy, tuberculosis, and malaria; Glivec patient assistance programs; and relief to support major humanitarian organisations with emergency medical needs.

PHARMACEUTICAL INDUSTRY IN INDIA

The pharmaceutical industry in India ranks 3rd in the world terms of volume and 14th in terms of value. According to the Department of Pharmaceuticals, Ministry of Chemicals and Fertilizers, the total turnover of India's pharmaceuticals industry between 2008 and September 2009 was US$21.04 billion. Hyderabad, Mumbai, Bangalore and Ahmedabad are the major pharmaceutical hubs of India. The domestic market was worth US$13.8 billion in 2013.The Government started to encourage the growth of drug manufacturing by Indian companies in the early 1960s, and with the Patents Act in 1970. However, economic liberalization in 90s by the former Prime Minister P.V. Narasimha Rao and the then Finance Minister, Dr. Manmohan Singh enabled the industry to become what it is today. This patent act removed composition patents from food and drugs, and though it kept process patents, these were shortened to a period of five to seven years.The Lack of patent protection made the Indian market undesirable to the multinational companies that had dominated the market. Whilst the multinationals streamed out, Indian companies carved a niche in both the Indian and world markets with their expertise in reverse-engineering new processes for manufacturing drugs at low costs. Although some of the larger companies have taken baby steps towards drug innovation, the industry as a whole has been following this business model until the present.India's biopharmaceutical industry clocked a 17 percent growth with revenues of Rs.137 billion ($3 billion) in the 2009-10 financial year over the previous fiscal. Bio-pharma was the biggest contributor generating 60 percent of the industry's growth at Rs.8,829 crore, followed by bio-services at Rs.2,639 crore and bio-agri at Rs.1,936 crore.

Overview

In 2002, over 20,000 registered drug manufacturers in India sold $9 billion worth of formulations and bulk drugs. 85% of these formulations were sold in India while over 60% of the bulk drugs were exported, mostly to the United States and Russia. Most of the players in the market are small-to-medium enterprises; 250 of the largest companies control 70% of the Indian market. Thanks to the 1970 Patent Act, multinationals represent only 35% of the market, down from 70% thirty years ago.

Most pharma companies operating in India, even the multinationals, employ Indians almost exclusively from the lowest ranks to high level management. Homegrown pharmaceuticals, like many other businesses in India, are often a mix of public and private enterprise.

In terms of the global market, India currently holds a modest 1–2% share, but it has been growing at approximately 10% per year. India gained its foothold on the global scene with its innovatively engineered generic drugs and active pharmaceutical ingredients (API), and it is now seeking to become a major player in outsourced clinical research as well as contract manufacturing and research. </ref>Indian companies received 304 Abbreviated New Drug Application (ANDA) approvals from the US Food and Drug Administration (USFDA) in 2017. The country accounts for around 30 per cent (by volume) and about 10 per cent (value) in the US$ 70-80 billion US generics market. Growth in other fields notwithstanding, generics are still a large part of the picture. India is the largest provider of generic drugs globally. Indian pharmaceutical sector industry supplies over 50 per cent of global demand for various vaccines, 40 per cent of generic demand in the US and 25 per cent of all medicine in UK.

Quality

Between 2015 and 2017, there were 31 FDA warning letters to Indian pharmaceutical companies citing serious Data Integrity issues, including data deletion, manipulation or fabrication of test results, see "An Analysis Of 2017 FDA Warning Letters On Data Integrity" By Barbara Unger, Unger Consulting Inc. According to Outsourcing Pharma in 2012 75% of counterfeit drugs supplied world over had some origins in India, followed by 7% from Egypt and 6% from China.

The Central Drug Standards Control Organisation (CDSCO), the drug regulatory authority of India conducted a nationwide survey in 2009 and announced that of "24,000 samples [that] were collected from all over India and tested. It was found that only 11 samples or 0.046% were spurious." In 2017 a similar survey found 3.16% of the medicines sampled were substandard and 0.0245% were fake. Those more commonly prescribed are probably more often faked.

Exports

Exports of pharmaceuticals products from India increased from US$6.23 billion in 2006-07 to US$8.7 billion in 2008-09 a combined annual growth rate of 21.25%. Some of the major pharmaceutical firms include Sun Pharmaceutical, Cadila Healthcare and Piramal Enterprises.

Patents

A significant change in intellectual property protection in India was the 1 January 2005 enactment of an amendment to India's patent law that reinstated product patents for the first time since 1972. The legislation took effect on the deadline set by the WTO's Trade-Related Aspects of Intellectual Property Rights (TRIPS) agreement, which mandated patent protection on both products and processes for a period of 20 years. Under this new law, India will be forced to recognise not only new patents but also any patents filed after 1 January 1995. In December 2005, the TRIPS pact was amended to incorporate specific safeguards to ensure that the public health concerns of affordability and accessibility for a large section of people in developing countries was not compromised. These amendments came into force only in January 2017, however, after two-thirds of the member countries ratified them. In the domestic market, this new patent legislation has resulted in fairly clear segmentation. The multinationals narrowed their focus onto high-end patents who make up only 12% of the market, taking advantage of their newly bestowed patent protection. Meanwhile, Indian firms have chosen to take their existing product portfolios and target semi-urban and rural populations.

Product Development

Indian companies are also starting to adapt their product development processes to the new environment. For years, firms have made their ways into the global market by researching generic competitors to patented drugs and following up with litigation to challenge the patent. This approach remains untouched by the new patent regime and looks to increase in the future. However, those that can afford it have set their sights on an even higher goal: new molecule discovery. Although the initial investment is huge, companies are lured by the promise of hefty profit margins and thus a legitimate competitor in the global industry. Local firms have slowly been investing more money into their R&D programs or have formed alliances to tap into these opportunities.

Small and Medium Enterprises

As promising as the future is for a whole, the outlook for small and medium enterprises (SME) is not as bright. The excise structure changed so that companies now have to pay a 16% tax on the maximum retail price (MRP) of their products, as opposed to on the ex-factory price. Consequently, larger companies cut back on outsourcing and what business is left shifted to companies with facilities in the four tax-free states – Himachal Pradesh, Jammu and Kashmir, Uttarakhand, and Jharkhand. Consequently, a large number of pharmaceutical manufacturers shifted their plant to these states, as it became almost impossible to continue operating in non-tax free zones. But in a matter of a couple of years the excise duty was revised on two occasions, first it was reduced to 8% and then to 4%. As a result, the benefits of shifting to a tax free zone was negated. This resulted in, factories in the tax free zones, to start up third-party manufacturing. Under this these factories produced goods under the brand names of other parties on job work basis.

As SMEs wrestled with the tax structure, they were also scrambling to meet the 1 July deadline for compliance with the revised Schedule M Good Manufacturing Practices (GMP). While this should be beneficial to consumers and the industry at large, SMEs have been finding it difficult to find the funds to upgrade their manufacturing plants, resulting in the closure of many facilities. Others invested the money to bring their facilities to compliance, but these operations were located in non-tax-free states, making it difficult to compete in the wake of the new excise tax. Swas Medicare is one of the small scale leading pharmaceutical company of India, which is owned and founded by a Physician.

Largest Companies

Sales, marketing, and business

Multinational Pharmaceutical Companies ranked as per active presence of sales, marketing and business in India

1. Pfizer
2. GlaxoSmithKline
3. Sanofi Aventis
4. Merck

The Indian biotech sector parallels that of the US in many ways. Both are filled with small start-ups while the majority of the market is controlled by a few powerful companies. Both are dependent upon government grants and venture capitalists for funding because neither will be commercially viable for years.

Pharmaceutical companies in both countries see growth potential in biotechnology and have either invested in existing start-ups or ventured into the field themselves.

Government Support

The Indian government established the Department of Biotechnology in 1986 under the Ministry of Science and Technology. Since then, there have been a number of dispensations offered by both the central government and various states to encourage the growth of the industry. India's science minister launched a program that provides tax incentives and grants for biotech start-ups and firms seeking to expand and establishes the Biotechnology Parks Society of India to support ten biotech parks by 2010. Previously limited to rodents, animal testing was expanded to include large animals as part of the minister's initiative. States have started to vie with one another for biotech business, and they are offering such goodies as exemption from VAT and other fees, financial assistance with patents and subsidies on everything ranging from investment to land to utilities.

The biotechnology sector faces some major challenges in its quest for growth. Chief among them is a lack of funding, particularly for firms that are just starting out. The most likely sources of funds are government grants and venture capital, which is a relatively young industry in India. Government grants are difficult to secure, and due to the expensive and uncertain nature of biotech research, venture capitalists are reluctant to invest in firms that have not yet developed a commercially viable product.

The government has addressed the problem of educated but unqualified candidates in its Draft National Biotech Development Strategy. This plan included a proposal to create a National Task Force that will work with the biotech industry to revise the curriculum for undergraduate and graduate study in life sciences and biotechnology. The government's strategy also stated intentions to increase the number of PhD Fellowships awarded by the Department of Biotechnology to 200 per year. These human resources will be further leveraged with a "Bio-Edu-Grid" that will knit together the resources of the academic and scientific industrial communities, much as they are in the US.

In 2019 the Department of Pharmaceuticals announced that as part of the Made in India initiative, drugs for local use must have 75% of local content, and drugs for export 10%. A bill of material must be produced for checking.

Foreign Investment

An initiative passed earlier this year allowed 100% foreign direct investment in the biotech sector without compulsory licensing from the government.

Pharmaceutical policy

Pharmaceutical policy is a branch of health policy that deals with the development, provision and use of medications within a health care system. It embraces drugs (both brand name and generic), biologics (products derived from living sources, as opposed to chemical compositions), vaccines and natural health products. Pharmaceutical policy includes:

Funding of Research in the Life Sciences

In many countries, an agency of the national government (in the U.S. the NIH, in the U.K. the MRC, and in India the DST) funds university researchers to study the causes of disease, which in some cases leads to the development of discoveries which can be transferred to pharmaceutical companies and biotechnology companies as a basis for drug development. By setting its budget, its research priorities and making decisions about which researchers to fund, there can be a significant impact on the rate of new drug development and on the disease areas in which new drugs are developed. For example, a major investment by the NIH into research on HIV in the 1980s certainly could be viewed as an important foundation for the many antiviral drugs that have subsequently been developed.

PATENT LAW

While patent laws are written to apply to all inventions, whether mechanical, pharmaceutical, or electronic, the interpretations of patent law made by government patent granting agencies (the United States Patent and Trademark Office, for example) and courts, can be very subject-matter specific with significant impact on the incentives for drug development and the availability of lower-priced generic drugs. For example, a recent decision by the United States Court of Appeals for the Federal Circuit in Pfizer v. Apotex, 480 F.3d 1348 (Fed.Cir.2007), held invalid a patent on the "pharmaceutical salt" formulation of a previously patented active ingredient. If that decision is not overturned by the United States Supreme Court, generic versions of the drug in controversy, Norvasc (amlodipine besylate) will be available much earlier. If the reasoning of the Federal Circuit in the case is applied more generally to other patents on pharmaceutical formulations, it would have a significant impact in speeding generic drug availability (and, conversely, some negative impact on the incentives and funding for the research and development of new drugs).

Licensing

This involves the approval of a product for sale in a jurisdiction. Typically a national agency such as the US Food and Drug Administration (specifically, the Center for Drug Evaluation and Research, or CDER), the UK Medicines and Healthcare Products Regulatory Agency or Health Canada or Ukrainian Drug Registration Agency is responsible for reviewing a product and approving it for sale. The regulatory process typically focuses on quality, safety and efficacy. To be approved for sale a product must demonstrate that it is generally safe (or has a favourable risk/benefit profile relative to the condition it is intended to treat), that it does what the manufacturer claims and that it is produced to high standards. Internal staff and expert advisory committees review products. Once approved, a product is given an approval letter or issued with a notice of compliance, indicating that it may now be sold in the jurisdiction. In some cases, such approvals may have conditions attached, requiring, for example additional 'post-marketing' trials to clarify an issue (such as efficacy in certain patient populations or interactions with other products) or criteria limiting the product to certain uses.

Pricing

In many jurisdictions drug prices are regulated. For example, in the UK the Pharmaceutical Price Regulation Scheme is intended to ensure that the National Health Service is able to purchase drugs at "reasonable prices." In Canada, the Patented Medicine Prices Review Board examines drug pricing, compares the proposed Canadian price to that of seven other countries and determines if a price is "excessive" or not. In these circumstances, drug manufacturers must submit a proposed price to the appropriate regulatory agency.

Reimbursement

Once a regulatory agency has determined the clinical benefit and safety of a product and pricing has been confirmed (if necessary), a drug manufacturer will typically submit it for evaluation by a payer of some sort. Payers may be private insurance plans, governments (through the provision of benefits plans to insured populations or specialized entities like Cancer Care Ontario, which funds in-hospital oncology drugs) or health care organizations such as hospitals. At this point the critical issue is cost-effectiveness. This is where the discipline of pharmaco-economics is often applied. This is a specialized field of health economics that looks at the cost/benefit of a product in terms of quality of life, alternative treatments (drug and non-drug) and cost reduction or avoidance in other parts of the health care system (for example, a drug may reduce the need for a surgical intervention, thereby saving money). Structures like the UK's National Institute for Health and Clinical Excellence and Canada's Common Drug Review evaluate products in this way. Some jurisdictions do not, however, evaluate products for cost-effectiveness. In some instances, individual drug benefit plans (or their administrators) may also evaluate products. Additionally, hospitals may have their own review committees (often called a Pharmacy and Therapeutics (P&T) committee) to make decisions about which drugs to fund from the hospital budget.

Drug plan administrators may also apply their own pricing rules outside of that set by national pricing agencies. For example, British Columbia uses a pricing model called reference-based pricing to set the price of drugs in certain classes. Many US pharmacy benefit managers (PBMs) use strategies like tiered formularies and preferred listings to encourage competition and downward pricing pressure, resulting in lower prices for benefits plans. Competitive procurement of this sort is common among large purchasers such as the US Veteran's Health Administration.

Typically, a manufacturer will provide an estimate of the projected use of a drug as well as the expected fiscal impact on a drug plan's budget. If necessary, a drug plan may negotiate a risk-sharing agreement to mitigate the potential for an unexpectedly large budget impact due to incorrect assumptions and projections.

Because the clinical trials used to generate information to support drug licensing are limited in scope and duration, drug plans may request ongoing post-market trials (often called Phase IV or pragmatic clinical trials) to demonstrate a product's 'real world safety and effectiveness.' These may take the form of a patient registry or other means of data collection and analysis.

Once a product is deemed cost-effective, a price negotiated (or applied in the case of a pricing model) and any risk-sharing agreement negotiated, the drug is placed on a drug list or formulary. Prescribers may choose drugs on the list for their patients, subject to any conditions or patient criteria.

FORMULARY MANAGEMENT

At the core of most reimbursement regimes is the drug list, or formulary. Managing this list can involve many different approaches. Negative lists – products that are not reimbursed under any circumstances are used in some jurisdictions (c.f. Germany). More dynamic formularies may have graduated listings such as Ontario's recent conditional listing model. As mentioned, formularies may be used to drive choice to lower cost drugs by structuring a sliding scale of co-payments favouring cheaper products or those for which there is a preferential agreement with the manufacturer. This is the principle underlying preferred drug lists used in many US state Medicaid programs. Some jurisdictions and plans (such as Italy) may also categorize drugs according to their 'essentialness' and determine the level of reimbursement the plan will provide and the portion that the patient is expected to pay.

Formularies may also segment drugs into categories for which a prior authorization is needed. This is usually done to limit the use of a high cost drug or one that has potential for inappropriate use (sometimes called 'off-label' as it involves using a product to treat conditions other than those for which its license was granted). In this circumstance a health care provider would have to seek permission to prescribe the product or the pharmacist would have to obtain permission prior to dispensing it.

Eligibility

Depending on the structure of the health care system, drugs may be purchased by patients themselves, a health care organization on behalf of patients or an insurance plan (public or private). Hospitals typically limit eligibility to their in-patients. Private plans may be employer-sponsored such as Blue Cross, mandated by legislation, as in Quebec or consist of an outsourcing arrangement for a public plan, such as the US Medicare Part D scheme. Public plans may be structured in a variety of ways including:

1. Universal, as in Australia's Pharmaceutical Benefits Scheme
2. Restricted by age, as in the Ontario Drug Benefit Plan for seniors
3. Segmented by disease group, such as Manitoba's cystic fibrosis drug plan
4. Geared to income, such as US Medicaid programs in many states

Additionally, plans may be structured to respond to the 'catastrophic' impact of drug expenses incurred by those with serious diseases or high drug spending relative to income. These patient populations, often called 'medically needy,' may have all or part of their drug costs covered by 'plans of last resort,' (typically government-sponsored). One such plan is Ontario's Trillium Drug Program.

Pharmaceutical policy may also be used to respond to health crises. For example, Argentina launched REMEDIAR during its financial crisis of 2002. The government-sponsored program provides a specified list of essential drugs to primary care clinics in low-income neighbourhoods. Similarly, Brazil provides drugs for HIV/AIDS free to all citizens as a deliberate public health policy choice. Eligibility policy also focuses on cost-sharing between a plan and the beneficiary (the insured person). Co-payments may be used to drive certain prescribing choices (for example, favouring generic over brand drugs or preferred over non-preferred products). Deductibles may be used as part of geared to income plans.

Prescribing

Pharmaceutical policy may also attempt to shape and inform prescribing. Prescribing may be limited to physicians or include certain classes of health care providers such as nurse practitioners and pharmacists. There may be limitations placed on each class of provider. This may take the form of prescribing criteria for a drug, limiting its prescribing to a particular type of specialist physician for example (such as HIV/AIDS drugs to physicians with advanced training in this area), or it may involve special drug lists that a specific type of health care provider (such as a nurse practitioner) may prescribe from.

Plans may also seek to influence prescribing by providing information to prescribers. This practice is often called 'academic detailing' to differentiate it from the detailing (provision of drug information) done by pharmaceutical companies. Organizations such as Australia's National Prescribing Service typify this technique, providing independent information, including head-to-head comparisons and cost-effectiveness information to prescribers to influence their choices. Additionally, efforts to promote the 'appropriate use' of medications may also involve other providers like pharmacists providing clinical consulting services. In settings such as hospitals and long-term care, pharmacists often collaborate closely with physicians to ensure optimal prescribing choices are made. In some jurisdictions, such as

Australia, pharmacists are compensated for providing medication reviews for patients outside of acute or long-term care settings. Pharmacist collaboration with family physicians in order to improve prescribing may also be funded.

Pharmacy Services

Pharmaceutical policy may also encompass how drugs are provided to beneficiaries. This includes the mechanics of drug distribution and dispensing as well as the funding of such services. For example, some HMOs in the US use a 'central fill' approach where all prescriptions are packaged and shipped from a central location instead of at a community pharmacy. In other jurisdictions, retail pharmacies are compensated for dispensing drugs to eligible beneficiaries. A state-operated approach may also be taken, as with Sweden's Apoteket, which had the monopoly on retail pharmacy until 2009, and was not-for-profit. Pharmaceutical policy may also subsidize smaller, more marginal pharmacies, using the rationale that they are needed health care providers. The UK's Essential Small Pharmacies Scheme works this way.

History of Marketing

According to etymologists, the term 'marketing' first appeared in dictionaries in the sixteenth century where it referred to the process of buying and selling at a market. The contemporary definition of 'marketing' as a process of moving goods from producer to consumer with an emphasis on sales and advertising first appeared in dictionaries in 1897.The term, marketing, is a derivation of the Latin word, mercatus meaning market-place or merchant.

Marketing History: an overview

In pre-literate societies, the distinctive shape of amphora served some of the functions of a label, communicating information about region of origin, the name of the producer and may have carried product quality claims

Historians of marketing tend to fall into two distinct branches of marketing history - the history of marketing practice and the history of marketing thought. These branches are often deeply divided and have very different roots. The history of marketing practice is grounded in the management and marketing disciplines, while the history of marketing thought is grounded in economic and cultural history. This means that the two branches ask very different types of research questions and employ different research tools and frameworks.

Historians of marketing have undertaken considerable investigation into the emergence of marketing practice, yet there is little agreement about when marketing first began. Some researchers argue that marketing practices can be found in antiquity while others suggest that marketing, in its modern form, emerged in conjunction with the rise of consumer culture in seventeenth and eighteenth century Europe while yet other researchers suggest that modern marketing was only fully realised in the decades following the industrial revolution in Britain from where it subsequently spread to Europe and North America. Hollander and others have suggested that the different dates for the emergence of marketing can be explained by problems surrounding the way that marketing has been defined - whether reference to 'modern marketing' as a planned, programmed repertoire of professional practice including activities such as segmentation, product differentiation, positioning and marketing communications versus 'marketing' as a simple form distribution and exchange.

Marketing in the Middle Ages

Market scene by Pieter Aertsen, c.1550

In England and Europe during the Middle Ages, market towns sprang up. Some analysts have suggested that the term, 'marketing,' may have first been used in the context of market towns where the term 'marketing' may have been used by producers to describe the process of carting and selling their produce and wares in market towns. Blintiff has investigated the early Medieval networks of market towns and suggests that by the 12th century there was an upsurge in the number of market towns and the emergence of merchant circuits as traders bulked up surpluses from smaller regional, different day markets and resold them at the larger centralised market towns.

Braudel and Reynold have made a systematic study of these European market towns between the thirteenth and fifteenth century. Their investigation shows that in regional districts markets were held once or twice a week, while daily markets were more common in the larger cities and towns. Over time, permanent shops began to open daily and gradually supplanted the periodic markets. Peddlers filled in the gaps in distribution by travelling door-to-door in order to sell produce and wares. The physical market was characterised by transactional exchange, bartering systems were commonplace and the economy was characterised by local trading. Braudel reports that, in 1600, goods travelled relatively short distances - grain 5–10 miles; cattle 40–70 miles; wool and wollen cloth 20–40 miles. However, following the European age of discovery, goods were imported from afar - calico cloth from India, porcelain, silk and tea from China, spices from India and South-East Asia and tobacco, sugar, rum and coffee from the New World.

Bronze plate for printing an advertisement for the Liu family needle shop at Jinan, Song dynasty China. It is considered the world's earliest identified printed advertising medium.

Although the rise of consumer culture and marketing in Britain and Europe have been studied extensively, less is known about developments elsewhere. Nevertheless, recent research suggests that China exhibited a rich history of early marketing practices; including branding, packaging, advertising and retail signage.

From as early as 200 BCE, Chinese packaging and branding was used to signal family, place names and product quality, and the use of government imposed product branding was used between 600 and 900 AD. Eckhart and Bengtsson have argued that during the Song Dynasty (960–1127), Chinese society developed a consumerist culture, where a high level of consumption was attainable for a wide variety of ordinary consumers rather than just the elite (p. 212). The rise of a consumer culture led to the commercial investment in carefully managed company image, retail signage, symbolic brands, trademark protection and the brand concepts of baoji, hao, lei, gongpin, piazi and pinpai, which roughly equate with Western concepts of family status, quality grading, and upholding traditional Chinese values (p. 219). Eckhardt and Bengtsson's analysis suggests that brands emerged in China as a result of the social needs and tensions implicit in consumer culture, in which brands provide social status and stratification. Thus, the evolution of brands in China stands in sharp contrast to the West where manufacturers pushed brands onto the market in order to differentiate, increase market share and ultimately profits (pp 218–219).

Marketing in Seventeenth and Eighteenth Century Europe

Josiah Wedgewood's 18th century techniques exhibited many of the characteristics of modern marketing

Scholars have identified specific instances of marketing practices in England and Europe in the seventeenth and eighteenth centuries. As trade between countries or regions grew, companies required information on which to base business decisions. Individuals and companies carried out formal and informal research on trade conditions. As early as 1380, Johann Fugger travelled from Augsburg to Graben in order to gather information on the international textile industry. He exchanged detailed letters on trade conditions in relevant areas. In the early 1700s British industrial houses were demanding information, that could be used for business decisions. In the early 18th-century, Daniel Defoe, a London merchant, published information on trade and economic resources of England and Scotland. Defoe was a prolific publisher and among his many publications are titles devoted to trade including; Trade of Britain Stated, 1707; Trade of Scotland with France, 1713 and The Trade to India Critically and Calmly Considered, 1720; all books that were highly popular with merchants and business houses of the period. While such activities might now be recognised as marketing research, at that time they were known as 'commercial research' or 'commercial intelligence' and not seen as part of the repertoire of activities that make up contemporary marketing practice.

Other scholars have found evidence of advertising and promotion in eighteenth century France and Italy as well as Britain. Far from being primitive efforts, early advertising showed a high level of sophistication in its execution and abilility to reach mass audiences. In a major review of consumer society, McKendrick, Brewer and Plumb found extensive evidence of eighteenth century English entrepreneurs using 'modern' marketing techniques, including product differentiation, sales promotion and loss leader pricing.

English industrialists, Josiah Wedgewood and Matthew Boulton, are often portrayed as pioneers of modern mass marketing methods. Wedgewood was known to have used marketing techniques such as direct mail, travelling salesmen and catalogues in the eighteenth century. Josiah Wedgewood's marketing was highly sophisticated and recognisably 'modern' in that he planned production with the sale in mind. He carried out serious investigations into the fixed and variable costs of production and recognised that increased production would lead to lower unit costs. He also inferred that selling at lower prices would lead to higher demand and recognised the value of achieving scale economies in production. By cutting costs and lowering prices, Wedgewood was able to generate higher overall profits. Similarly, one of Wedgewood's contemporaries, Matthew Boulton, pioneered early mass production techniques and product differentiation at his Soho Manufactory in the 1760s. He also practiced planned obsolescence and understood the importance of 'celebrity marketing' - that is supplying the nobility, often at prices below cost and of obtaining royal patronage, for the sake of the publicity and cudos generated.

Fullerton argues that the practice of market segmentation emerged well before marketers used the notion formally. Certain strands of evidence suggest that simple examples of market segmentation were evident prior to the 1880s. The business historian, Richard S. Tedlow, argues that any attempt to segment markets prior to 1880 was highly fragmented since the economy was characterised by small, regional suppliers who mostly sold goods on a local or regional basis. When retail shops began to appear from the 15th century, retailers needed to separate the "riff raff" from wealthier customers. Outside the major metropolitan cities, few stores could afford to serve one type of clientele exclusively. However, gradually retail shops introduced innovations that would allow them to separate wealthier customers from the lower classes and peasants. One technique was to have a window opening out onto the street from which customers could be served. This allowed the sale of goods to the common people, without encouraging them to come inside. Another solution, that came into vogue from the late sixteenth century was to invite favoured customers into a back-room of the store, where goods were permanently on display. Yet another technique that emerged around the same time was to hold a showcase of goods in the shopkeeper's private home for the benefit of wealthier clients. Samuel Pepys, for example, writing in 1660, describes being invited to the home of a retailer to view a wooden jack. The eighteenth century English entrepreneurs, Josiah Wedgewood and Matthew Boulton, both staged expansive showcases of their wares in their private residences or in rented halls. Evidence of early marketing segmentation has also been noted across Europe. A study of the German book trade found examples of both product differentiation and market segmentation in the 1820s.

Marketing in the Nineteenth and Twentieth Centuries

Henry Ford began manufacturing the mass-produced Model T in 1908. Ford famously said that customers could own a car in any colour as long as it was black.

Until the nineteenth century, Western economies were characterised by small regional suppliers who sold goods on a local or regional basis. However, as transportation systems improved from the mid nineteenth century, the economy became more unified allowing companies to distribute standardised, branded goods a national level. This gave rise to a much broader mass marketing mindset. Manufacturers tended to insist on strict standardisation in order to achieve scale economies with a view to keeping production costs down and also to achieving market penetration in the early stages of a product's life cycle. The Model T Ford was an example of a product being manufactured at a price that was affordable for the burgeoning middle classes.

In the early twentieth century, as market size increased, it became more commonplace for manufacturers to produce a variety of models pitched at different quality points designed to meet the needs of various demographic and lifestyle market segments, giving rise to the widespread practice of market segmentation and product differentation. Between 1902 -1910 George B Waldron, working at Mahin's advertising agency, used tax registers, city directories and census data to show advertisers the proportion of educated versus illiterate consumers and the earning capacity of different occupations in what is believed to be the first example of demographic segmentation of a population. Within little more than a decade, Paul Cherington had developed the 'ABCD' household typology - the first socio-demographic segmentation tool. By the 1930s, market researchers such as Ernest Dichter were carrying out qualitative research into brand purchasers realised that demographic factors alone were insufficient to explain different marketing behaviour of various user groups. This insight led to the exploration of other factors such as lifestyles, values, attitudes and beliefs in market segmentation and advertising.

When Wendell R. Smith published his now classic article, Product Differentiation and Market Segmentation as Alternative Marketing Strategies in 1956, he noted that he was simply documenting marketing practices that had been observed for some time and which he described as a "natural force". Other theorists agree that Smith was simply codifying implicit knowledge that had been used in marketing and brand management from the early twentieth century.

As industry grew, the demand for skilled business professionals also grew. To meet this demand, universities began offering courses in commerce, economics and marketing. Marketing, as a discipline, was first taught in universities in the very early twentieth century.However, researchers only became interested in investigating the history of marketing in the mid twentieth century. From the outset, researchers tended to identify two strands of historical research; the history of marketing practice and the history of marketing thought which was fundamentally concerned with the rise of marketing education and dissecting the way that marketing was taught and studied.Early historical studies were primarily descriptive.

History of Marketing Practice

The practice of marketing may have been carried out for millennia, but the modern concept of marketing as a professional practice appears to have emerged the post industrial corporate world. In addition to the studies of specific cultures or time periods, discussed in the preceding section, some historians of marketing have sought to write more general histories of marketing's evolution in the modern era. A key question that has preoccupied researchers is whether it is possible to identify specific orientations or mindsets that inform key periods in marketing's evolution. Marketers disagree about the way that marketing practice has evolved over time.

Orientations and Philosophies

In the marketing literature, continuing debate surrounds the orientations or philosophies that might have informed marketing practice at different periods of time. An orientation may be defined as "the type of activity or subject that an organisation seems most interested in and gives most attention to". In relation to marketing orientations, the term has been defined as a "philosophy of business management". or "a corporate state of mind" or as an "organisational culture".

Common Periods

The general lack of agreement amongst scholars as to what constitutes clearly identifiable periods and the orientation that characterised each distinct period has spawned a lengthy list of orientations. Space prevents an exhaustive description of all periods or eras. However, the salient features of the most commonly cited periods appear in the following section.

Production Orientation

A production orientation is often proposed as the first of the so-called orientations that dominated business thought. Keith dated the production era from the 1860s to the 1930s, but other theorists argue that evidence of the production orientation can still be found in some companies or industries. Specifically Kotler and Armstrong note that the production philosophy is "one of the oldest philosophies that guides sellers" and "is still useful in some situations".

The production orientation is characterised by:

- Focus on production, manufacturing, and efficiency
- Attainment of economies of scale, economies of scope, experience effects or all three
- Assumption that demand exceeds supply
- Mindset that is encapsulated by Say's Law; "Supply creates its own demand" or "if somebody makes a product, somebody else will want to buy it"

- Limited research that is largely limited to technical-product research rather than customer research
- Rose to prominence in an environment which had a shortage of manufactured goods relative to demand, so goods sold easily.
- Minimal promotion and advertising, marketing communications limited to raising awareness of the product's existence

Selling Orientation

The sales orientation, often characterised by door-to-door selling is thought to have begun during the Great Depression of the 1890s and continues to this day. Pictured: A Rawleigh's salesman in 1915

The selling orientation is thought to have begun during the Great Depression and continued well into the 1950s although examples of this orientation can still be found today. Kotler et al. note that the selling concept "is typically practised with unsought goods".

The selling orientation is characterised by:

- Aggressive selling to push products, often involving door-to-door selling
- Accepting every possible sale or booking, regardless of its suitability for the business
- Strong transactional focus (ignores potential relationships)

Marketing Orientation

The marketing orientation or the marketing concept emerged in the 1950s. Characteristics of the marketing orientation:

- Thorough understanding of the customer's needs, wants and behaviors should be the focal point of all marketing decisions
- Marketing efforts (sales, advertising, product management, pricing) should be integrated and in tune with the customer
- New product concepts should flow from extensive market analysis and product testing

SOCIETAL MARKETING CONCEPT

Phillip Kotler is often credited with first proposing the societal marketing orientation or concept in an article published in the Harvard Business Review in 1972. However, some marketing historians, notably Wilkie and Moore, have argued that a societal perspective was evident in marketing theory and in marketing texts, since the discipline's inception in the early 1900s or that societal marketing is merely an extension of the marketing concept.

The societal marketing concept adopts the position that marketers have a greater social responsibility than simply satisfying customers and providing them with superior value. Instead, marketing activities should strive to benefit society's overall well-being. Marketing organisations that have embraced the societal marketing concept typically identify key stakeholder groups including: employees, customers, local communities, the wider public and government and consider the impact of their activities on all stakeholders. They ensure that marketing activities do not damage the environment and are not hazardous to broader society. Societal marketing developed into sustainable marketing.

Characteristics of societal marketing:

- An attempt to balance corporate commitments to groups and individuals in its environment, including customers, other businesses, employees and investors.
- Companies must include social and ethical considerations into their marketing practices
- Consideration is given to the environment includes problems such as air, water, and land pollution
- Consideration is given to consumer rights, unfair pricing and ethics in advertising

Relationship Orientation

Starting in the 1990s, a new stage of marketing emerged called relationship marketing. The focus of relationship marketing is on a long-term relationship that benefits both the company and the customer. The relationship is based on trust and commitment, and both companies tend to shift their operating activities to be able to work more efficiently together. One of the most prominent reasons for relationship marketing comes from Kotler's idea that it costs about five times more to obtain a new customer than to maintain the relationship with an existing customer. A relationship marketing approach seeks to maximise the value of all the potential exchanges an organisation could have into the future.

The characteristics of relationship marketing include:

- Focus on the relationship between seller and buyer
- Investment in the lifetime of relationships rather than single transactions by calculating customer lifetime value (CLV)
- Orientation on product benefits and/or customer value
- Better customer service, commitment, and contact
- Quality is the concern of all
- All activities are coordinated with the customer interface, including the customer's involvement in the firm's processes
- Customised offerings where practical

Empirical support for relationship marketing as a distinct paradigm is very weak. One study suggests that relationship marketing is really a sub-component of large scale movements of the value-added process rather than a separate era or framework. Some theorists suggest that marketing is moving from a relationship marketing paradigm and towards a social media paradigm where marketers have access to a more controlled environment and are able to customise offers and communications messages.

Periodisations

To investigate the history of marketing practice, scholars often turn to a method known as periodisation. Periodisation refers to the process or study of categorizing the past into discrete, quantified, named units for the purpose of analysis or study. Scholars do not agree on the periods that characterise the history of marketing practice. In a major review of the periodisation approach, Hollander et al. have identified fourteen different "stage theories" or "short periodisations" as well as a total of nineteen "long periodisations" that have been carried out since 1957. Of these, the contributions of Robert Keith (1960) and Ronald Fullerton (1988) are the most frequently cited.

Keith's Periodisation

In 1960, Robert Keith, the then Vice President of Pillsbury, set the stage for decades of controversy when he published an article entitled the "Marketing Revolution" in which he set out the way that the Pillsbury Company had shifted from a focus on production in the 1860s through to a consumer focus in the 1950s. He traced three distinct eras in Pillsbury's evolution:

- Production-oriented era (1869–1930s): characterised by a "focus on production processes"
- Sales-oriented era (1930s–1950s): characterised by investment in research to develop new products and advertising to persuade markets of product benefits
- Marketing-oriented era (1950s–present): characterised by a focus on the customer's latent and existing needs

In addition, Keith hypothesised that a "marketing control era" was about to emerge. Although Keith's article explicitly documented Pillsbury's evolution, the article appears to suggest that the stages observed at Pillsbury constitute a standard or normal evolutionary path (production'! sales'! marketing) for most large organisations.

Keith's notion of distinct eras in the evolution of marketing practice has been widely criticised and his periodisation described as "hopelessly flawed". Specific criticisms of Keith's tripartite periodisation include that:

- It ignores historical facts about business conditions
- It misstates the nature of supply and demand

- It slights the growth of marketing institutions

The article, which is entirely based on Keith's personal recollections and did not use a single reference, is best described as anecdotal. Systematic studies carried out since Keith's work have failed to replicate Keith's periodisation. Instead, other studies suggest that many companies exhibited a marketing orientation in the 19th-century and that the business schools were teaching marketing decades before Pillsbury adopted a marketing-oriented approach. Jones and Richardson also investigated historical accounts of marketing practice and found evidence for both the sales and marketing era during the so-called production era and concluded that there was no "marketing revolution". A detailed study of the chocolate manufacturer, Rowntree, found that this company had shifted from a production orientation through to a marketing orientation by the 1930s, without having transitioned through the so-called sales orientation. Other critiques of Keith's work have pointed out that the so-called "production era" fails to align with historical facts and have suggested that it is a myth. Keith's eras have become known, somewhat cynically, as the standard chronology.

Fullerton's Periodisation

The English industrial revolution is often seen as a trigger for the rise of modern marketing

In 1988, Fullerton developed a more subtle and nuanced periodisation for the so-called marketing eras. Fullerton's eras were:

- Era of antecedents (1500–1750): a long gestational period in which people were largely self-sufficient and rural; economy characterised by low levels of consumption; commerce was seen as suspicious
- Era of origins (1750–1870): precipitated by the dislocations of the English industrial revolution and the rise of a more urban population, this era is characterised by more attention to persuasive tactics designed to stimulate demand
- Era of institutional development (1850–1929): many of the large institutions and modern marketing practices emerged during this period
- Era of refinement and formalization (1930–present): further development and refinement of principles and practices developed in the preceding period

In spite of the intense criticism leveled at Keith's eras of marketing practice, his periodisation is the most frequently cited in textbooks and has become the accepted wisdom. One content analysis of 25 introductory and advanced texts found that Keith's eras were reproduced in all but four. Another study, which examined 15 of the top selling marketing texts, found that the although the incidence of repeating

Keith's eras was waning, it had not been replaced by Fullerton's periodisation, nor any other more meaningful framework.

Other Periodisations

For all the controversies surrounding marketing stages or periods, Keith and others appear to have contributed a lasting legacy. A study by Grundey (2010) suggests that many contemporary textbooks begin with Keith's eras and expand on it by including newer concepts such as the societal marketing concept, the relationship marketing concept and the interfunctional concept, as shown in the table below. More recently, Kotler and Keller added the holistic marketing concept to the list of eras in marketing. Marketing theorists continue to debate whether the holistic era represents a genuine new orientation or whether it is an extension of the marketing concept. Grundey summarised five different periodisations in the history of marketing, as shown in the following table, as a means of highlighting the general lack of agreement among scholars.

HISTORY OF MARKETING THOUGHT

University of Pennsylvania was among the first universities to offer courses in marketing Dating the history of marketing, as an academic discipline, is just as problematic as the history of marketing practice. Marketing historians cannot agree on how to date the beginnings of marketing thought. Eric Shaw, for instance, suggests that a period of pre-academic marketing thought can be identified prior to 1900. Other historians suggest that the theory of marketing only emerged in the 20th century when the discipline began to offer courses at universities. Nevertheless, the birth of marketing as a discipline is usually designated to the first decade of the twentieth century when "marketing courses" appeared in universities. In 1902, the University of Michigan offered what many believe to be the very first course in marketing. The University of Illinois also started offering coursework in marketing in 1902.In the academic year, 1904-1905, the University of Pennsylvania commenced teaching marketing. Other universities soon followed, including the Harvard Business School.

Prior to the emergence of marketing courses, marketing was not recognised as a discipline in its own right; rather it was treated as a branch of economics and was often called applied economics. Subjects, which today might be recognised as marketing-related, were embedded in economics courses. Early marketing theories were described as modifications or adaptations of economic theories.

The impetus for the separation of marketing and economics was due, at least in part, to economic's focus on production as the creator of economic value and general failure to investigate distribution. In the late 19th century and early 20th century, as markets became more globalised, distribution began to assume increasing importance. Some economics professors began to run courses examining various aspects of the marketing system, including "distributive and regulative systems." Other courses, such as the "marketing of products" and the "marketing of farm-products" followed. As the first decades of the 20th century progressed, books and articles concerning marketing topics began to emerge. In 1936, the publication of the new Journal of Marketing gave marketing academics a forum for exchanging ideas and research methods and also gave the discipline a real sense of its own distinct identity as a maturing academic discipline.

A periodisation Approach

Several scholars have attempted to describe the evolution of marketing thought chronologically and to connect it with broader intellectual and academic trends. Bartels (1965) provided a brief account of marketing's formative periods, and Shah and Gardner (1982) briefly considered the development of the six dominant schools in contemporary marketing. However, these initial attempts have been criticised as overly descriptive. One of the first theorists to consider the stages in the development of marketing thought was Robert Bartels, who in The History of Marketing Thought, (1965) used a periodisation approach. He categorised the development of marketing theory decade by decade from the beginning of the 20th century:

- 1900s: discovery of basic concepts and their exploration
- 1910s: conceptualisation, classification and definition of terms
- 1920s: integration on the basis of principles
- 1930s: development of specialisation and variation in theory
- 1940s: reappraisal in the light of new demands and a more scientific approach
- 1950s: reconceptualisation in the light of managerialism, social development and quantitative approaches
- 1960s: differentiation on bases such as managerialism, holism, environmentalism, systems, and internationalism
- 1970s: socialisation; the adaptation of marketing to social change

Bartels was the first historian to provide a "long view of marketing's past and wide sweep of its subdisciplines" and in so doing, he nurtured an interest in the history of marketing thought.

A 'SCHOOLS OF THOUGHT' APPROACH

Other marketing historians have eschewed the periodisation approach, and instead considered whether distinct schools within marketing reflect different facets of common theory and whether a more unifying intellectual structure has emerged. These approaches tend to identify distinct schools of thought. A school of thought refers to an intellectual tradition or a group of scholars who share a common philosophy or set of ideas. Marketing historians, Shaw and Jones, define a school of thought as one that has "a substantial body of knowledge; developed by a number of scholars; and describing at least one aspect of the what, how, who, why, when and where of performing marketing activities."

To a certain extent, there is some agreement that in early marketing thought, three so-called traditional schools, namely the commodity school, the functional school and the institutional school co-existed. Marketing historians such as Eric Shaw and Barton A. Weitz point to the publication of Wroe Alderson's book, Marketing Behavior and Executive Action (1957), as a break-point in the history of marketing thought, moving from the macro functions-institutions-commodities approach to a micromarketing managementparadigm. Following on from Alderson, marketing began to incorporate other fields of knowledge besides economics, notably behavioral science and psychology, becoming a multi-disciplinary field. For many scholars, Alderson's book marks the beginning of the Marketing Management Era. Of those historians who identify schools, there is no real agreement about which schools were dominant at different stages in marketing's development. Although the distinctive features of these schools can be identified and described, many of the early text-books included elements drawn from two or more schools of thought-for example, in a series of chapters devoted to commodities followed by a series of chapters devoted to the institutional and functional schools.

In the following section, a brief overview of the contributions of key thinkers will be outlined with respect to the prevailing schools that have dominated marketing thought.

Hunt and Goolsby, identified four schools of thought that have dominated marketing, namely; the commodity school, the institutional school, the functional school and the managerial school.

- The Commodity School: A focus on different types of goods in the market-place and how they are marketed.
- The Institutional School: Emphasised the functions of middlemen (or inter-mediaries); similar to the functional school, but with a focus on channel flows.
- The Functional School: A focus on the characteristics of marketing, identi-fying the functions and systems of marketing; adopts a systems approach.
- The Managerial School: A focus on the problems faced by marketing man-agers; focuses on the perspective of the seller.

Some marketing historians like Jagdish Sheth have identified the modern "marketing schools" as:

- The Managerial school emerged during the late 1950s and became argu-ably the predominant and most influential school of thought in the field
- The Consumer/buyer behavior school, which dominated the academic field in the second half of the twentieth century (apart from the Managerial school), features theories emerging from behavioral science

- The Social exchange school, which focuses on exchange as the fundamental concept of marketing

Yet other commentators identify a broader range of schools. O'Malley and Lichrou, for example, document the schools as:

- Functional: What activities does marketing perform? Focus on intermediaries and value adding.
- Commodities: How are goods classified? Focus on classification of goods; trade flows
- Marketing Institutions: Who performs marketing functions on commodities? Focus on retailers, wholesalers, intermediaries, distribution channels
- Marketing Management: How should marketers and managers market products and services to consumers? Business firm as seller/ supplier
- Marketing Systems: What is a marketing system and how does it work? Channels of distribution and aggregate systems,
- Consumer behaviour: How and why do consumers buy? organisational buyer and consumer buyer
- Macro-marketing: How do marketing systems impact on society? Industries, channels, consumer movement, environmentalism
- Exchange: What are the forms of exchange? Who are the parties to the exchange process? Aggregations of buyers and sellers
- Marketing history: When did marketing practice and ideas emerge and evolve? Marketing thought and marketing practice

Brief Description of the Dominant Schools of Thought

By the 1920s, the marketing discipline was organised into three schools of thought: the commodity school, the institutional school and the functional school.The following sections briefly outlines the schools of thought as conceptualised by key thinkers in the discipline. Although these can be treated as separate schools of thought, considerable overlap between them is evident. The three schools that preceded marketing management exhibited a highly descriptive approach and collectively these are often called the classical schools. These schools borrowed heavily from economics and were largely concerned with aggregate demand and lacked a focus on the individual firm. By the 1960s, all previous schools of thought had been eclipsed by the managerial school because it offered a problem-solving approach and presented marketers with potential solutions to marketing problems that were frequently encountered.

The Commodity School

The commodity school is thought to have originated with an article by C.C. Parlin (1916) with a focus on the objects of exchange and was primarily concerned with classifying commodities. A different article published by Copeland, and published in the Harvard Business Review(1923) proposed the convenience-shopping-specialty goods classification which is still in use today. Other theorists developed a plethora of methods for classifying goods.

The Institutional School

The institutional school focused its attention on the agents of market transactions, specifically those organisations active in the intermediary channel system, such as wholesalers and retailers. It was primarily concerned with documenting the channels of distribution, the functions performed by channel members and the value-adding services they provided. In short, the institutional school was fundamentally concerned with the activities required to achieve efficiency within distribution systems. The institutional school was heavily influenced by economics, but in the 1970s, began to take on ideas from behavioural science. A key work in the institutional school tradition is Weld's The Marketing of Farm Products, (1916) while other important contributors included: Butler's Marketing and Merchandising, (1923); Breyer's Commodity and Marketing (1931); Converse's Marketing: Methods and Policies (1921) and Duddy & Revzan's Marketing: An Institutional Approach(1947).

The Functional School

The functional school was thought to have originated with the publication of Shaw's article, Some Problems in Market Distribution, (1912) The functional school was primarily concerned with documenting the functions of marketing. In other words, it attempted to address the question, What work does marketing do? Different theorists within the functional school produced long lists of marketing's functions. Although there was little agreement about what should be included in the list, much of it revolved around the value added by marketing intermediaries. In those early years, advertising and promotion was rarely seen as a marketing function. In addition to Shaw, key thinkers in the functional school included Weld, Vanderblue and Ryan.

Marketing Management

The marketing management school focuses on typical problems encountered by marketers

Wroe Alderson changed marketing thought with the publication of his work, Marketing Behaviour and Executive Action (1957) in which he was primarily concerned with the problems and challenges faced by marketers and the types of solutions that had been found to be successful. This shifted the emphasis away from the functions of marketing and towards a more problem-solving approach, thereby paving the way for a more managerial approach within the discipline. Some historians have claimed that Alderson's article signalled a paradigm shift in thinking, towards a new macromarketing approach.

The marketing management school emerged as the dominant school in the 1960s following the publication of Basic Marketing: A Managerial Approach, written by E. Jerome McCarthy and replaced the so-called functional school which had been the dominant school for the first part of the twentieth century. In the words of Hunt and Goolsby, the publication of McCarthy's text, sounded the "beginning of the end for the functional school." However, Hunt and Goolsby note that the 1960s was a transitional period in which both the functional school and the managerial school co-existed. Shaw and Jones have described the emergence of the managerial school in the mid-twentieth century as a "paradigm shift."

While the management school continued to borrow from economics, it also introduced ideas from the new and emerging fields of sociology and psychology, which offered useful insights for explaining aspects of consumer behaviour such as the influence of culture and social class. Key works in the marketing management tradition include Wroe Alderson's Marketing Behavior and Executive Action, (1957), Howard's Marketing Management (1957), Lazer's Managerial Marketing: Perspectives and Viewpoints, (1957) and McCarthy's Basic Marketing: A Managerial Approach (1960).

The salient features of the managerial approach to marketing are:

- "an overt marketing-as-management orientation, and
- an overt reliance on the behavioral and quantitative sciences as means of knowing."

Key Innovations that Influenced Marketing Practice

- 1450: Gutenberg's metal movable type, leading eventually to mass-production of flyers and brochures
- 1600s: Paid advertising in Italy
- 1600s: Use of handbills and posters is common practice in Elizabethan England
- 1605: World's first newspaper published in Germany
- 1600s and 1700s: Posters and handbills used for promotion in England
- 1665: The Oxford Gazette first published in England (later renamed the London Gazette and still published today)
- 1700s: Widespread emergence of newspapers and magazines in England and France; by the 1730s daily newspapers in London devoted more than half the available space to advertising
- 1719: The Daily Post first published; early instance of a periodical dedicated to business, science and innovation
- 1836: Paid advertising in a newspaper (in France)

- 1839: Posters on private property banned in England

The telegraph was an early form of mass communication

- 1864: Earliest recorded use of the telegraph for mass unsolicited spam
- 1867: Earliest recorded billboard rentals
- 1876: Films produced by French film-makers, Auguste and Louis Lumiere, made at the request of a representative of Lever Brothers in France and feature Sunlight soap, are thought to be the first recorded instance of paid product placement.

Sunlight was an early advertiser in cinema, radio and TV. Pictured: Advertisement for Sunlight Soap washing powder, 1897

- 1880s: Early examples of trademarks as branding
- 1902: The first marketing course, taught by Edward David Jones, was offered at the University of Michigan
- 1905: The University of Pennsylvania offered a course in "The Marketing of Products"
- 1908: Harvard Business School opens - Harvard was an early influence on marketing thought
- 1920: The magazine, Variety, reports that 50% of cinemas show advertising programmes
- 1920s: Radio advertising commences
- 1940s: Electronic computers developed
- 1941: First recorded use of television advertising
- 1955: Television viewing exceeded radio listening for the first time in Britain
- 1950s: Systematization of telemarketing
- 1957: Three key scholarly texts published Wroe Alderson's Marketing Behavior and Executive Action; Howard's Marketing Managementand Lazer's Managerial Marketing: Perspectives and Viewpoints
- 1960 E. Jerome McCarthy published his now classic, Basic Marketing: A Managerial Approach (1960).
- 1970s: E-commerce developed
- 1980s: Development of database marketing as precursor to CRM
- 1980s: Emergence of relationship marketing
- 1980s: Emergence of computer-oriented spam
- 1984: Introduction of guerrilla tactics
- 1985: Desktop publishing democratises the production of print-advertising (precursor to consumer-generated media and content)

- 1991: IMC gains academic status
- Mid 1990s: Modern search engines started appearing in the mid-1990s, with Google making its debut in 1998
- 1990s CRM and IMC (in various guises and names) gain dominance in promotions and marketing planning,
- 1996: Identification of viral marketing
- 2000s: Integrated marketing gains widespread acceptance with its first dedicated academic research centre opened in 2002
- 2003 -2006: Emergence of social media. MySpace and LinkedIn emerged in 2003, Facebook in 2004 and Twitter in 2006.

Many countries have measures in place to limit advertising by pharmaceutical companies.

Pharmaceutical company spending on marketing far exceeds that of its research budget. In Canada, $1.7 billion was spent in 2004 to market drugs to physicians; in the United States, $21 billion was spent in 2002. In 2005, money spent on pharmaceutical marketing in the United States was estimated at $29.9 billion with one estimate as high as $57 billion. When the U.S. numbers are broken down, 56% was free samples, 25% was pharmaceutical sales representative "detailing" (promoting drugs directly to) physicians, 12.5% was direct to user advertising, 4% on detailing to hospitals, and 2% on journal ads. There is some evidence that marketing practices can negatively affect both patients and the health care profession.

To health Care Providers

Marketing to health-care providers takes three main forms: activity by pharmaceutical sales representatives, provision of drug samples, and sponsoring continuing medical education(CME). The use of gifts, including pens and coffee mugs embossed with pharmaceutical product names, has been prohibited by PHRMA ethics guidelines since 2008. Of the 237,000 medical sites representing 680,000 physicians surveyed in SK&A's 2010 Physician Access survey, half said they prefer or require an appointment to see a rep (up from 38.5% preferring or requiring an appointment in 2008), while 23% won't see reps at all, according to the survey data. Practices owned by hospitals or health systems are tougher to get into than private practices, since appointments have to go through headquarters, the survey found. 13.3% of offices with just one or two doctors won't see representatives, compared with a no-see rate of 42% at offices with 10 or more doctors. The most accessible physicians for promotional purposes are allergists/immunologists – only 4.2% won't see reps at all – followed by orthopedic specialists (5.1%) and diabetes specialists (7.6%). Diagnostic radiologists are the most rigid about allowing details – 92.1% won't see reps – followed by pathologists and neuroradiologists, at 92.1% and 91.8%, respectively.

E-detailing is widely used to reach "no see physicians"; approximately 23% of primary care physicians and 28% of specialists prefer computer-based edetailing, according to survey findings reported in the 25 April 2011, edition of American Medical News (AMNews), published by the American Medical Association (AMA).

PhRMA Code

The Pharmaceutical Research and Manufacturers of America (PhRMA) released updates to its voluntary Code on Interactions with Healthcare Professionals on 10 July 2008. The new guidelines took effect in January 2009."

In addition to prohibiting small gifts and reminder items such as pens, notepads, staplers, clipboards, paperweights, pill boxes, etc., the revised Code:

1. Prohibits company sales representatives providing restaurant meals to healthcare professionals, but allows them to provide occasional modest meals in healthcare professionals' offices in conjunction with informational presentations"
2. Includes new provisions requiring companies to ensure their representatives are sufficiently trained about applicable laws, regulations, and industry codes of practice and ethics.
3. Provides that each company will state its intentions to abide by the Code and that company CEOs and compliance officers will certify each year that they have processes in place to comply.
4. Includes more detailed standards regarding the independence of continuing medical education.
5. Provides additional guidance and restrictions for speaking and consulting arrangements with healthcare professionals.

Free samples

Free samples have been shown to affect physician prescribing behaviour. Physicians with access to free samples are more likely to prescribe brand name medication over equivalent generic medications. Other studies found that free samples decreased the likelihood that physicians would follow standard of care practices.

Receiving pharmaceutical samples does not reduce prescription costs. Even after receiving samples, sample recipients remain disproportionately burdened by prescription costs.

It is argued that a benefit to free samples is the "try it before you buy it" approach. Free samples give immediate access to the medication and the patient can begin treatment right away. Also, it saves time from going to a pharmacy to get it filled before treatment begins. Since not all medications work for everyone, and many do not work the same way for each person, free samples allow patients to find which dose and brand of medication works best before having to spend money on a filled prescription at a pharmacy.

Continuing medical Education

Hours spent by physicians in industry-supported continuing medical education (CME) is greater than that from either medical schools or professional societies.

Pharmaceutical Representatives

Currently, there are approximately 81,000 pharmaceutical sales representatives in the United States pursuing some 830,000 pharmaceutical prescribers. A pharmaceutical representative will often try to see a given physician every few weeks. Representatives often have a call list of about 200-300 physicians with 120-180 targets that should be visited in 1-2 or 3 week cycle.

Because of the large size of the pharmaceutical sales force, the organization, management, and measurement of effectiveness of the sales force are significant business challenges. Management tasks are usually broken down into the areas of physician targeting, sales force size and structure, sales force optimization, call planning, and sales forces effectiveness. A few pharmaceutical companies have realized that training sales representatives on high science alone is not enough, especially when most products are similar in quality. Thus, training sales representatives on relationship selling techniques in addition to medical science and product knowledge, can make a difference in sales force effectiveness. Specialist physicians are relying more and more on specialty sales reps for product information, because they are more knowledgeable than primary care reps.

The United States has 81,000 pharmaceutical representatives or 1 for every 7.9 physicians. The number and persistence of pharmaceutical representatives has placed a burden on the time of physicians. "As the number of reps went up, the amount of time an average rep spent with doctors went down—so far down, that tactical scaling has spawned a strategic crisis. Physicians no longer spend much time with sales reps, nor do they see this as a serious problem."

Marketers must decide on the appropriate size of a sales force needed to sell a particular portfolio of drugs to the target market. Factors influencing this decision are the optimal reach (how many physicians to see) and frequency (how often to see them) for each individual physician, how many patients suffer from that disease state, how many sales representatives to devote to office and group practice and how many to devote to hospital accounts if needed. To aid this decision, customers are broken down into different classes according to their prescription behavior, patient population, and of course, their business potential.

Marketers attempt to identify the set of physicians most likely to prescribe a given drug. Historically, this was done by measuring the number of total prescriptions (TRx) and new prescriptions (NRx) per week that each physician writes. This information is collected by commercial vendors. The physicians are then "deciled" into ten groups based on their writing patterns. Higher deciles are more aggressively targeted. Some pharmaceutical companies use additional information such as:

- Profitability of a prescription (script),
- Accessibility of the physician,
- Tendency of the physician to use the pharmaceutical company's drugs,
- Effect of managed care formularies on the ability of the physician to prescribe a drug,
- The adoption sequence of the physician (that is, how readily the physician adopts new drugs in place of older treatments), and
- The tendency of the physician to use a wide palette of drugs
- Influence that physicians have on their colleagues.

Physicians are perhaps the most important component in sales. They write the prescriptions that determine which drugs will be used by people. Influencing the physician is the key to pharmaceutical sales. Historically, this was done by a large pharmaceutical sales force. A medium-sized pharmaceutical company might have a sales force of 1000 representatives. The largest companies have tens of thousands of representatives around the world. Sales representatives called upon physicians regularly, providing clinical information, approved journal articles, and free drug samples. This is still the approach today; however, economic pressures on the industry are causing pharmaceutical companies to rethink the traditional sales process to physicians. The industry has seen a large scale adoption of Pharma CRM systems that works on laptops and more recently tablets. The new age pharmaceutical representative is armed with key data at his fingertips and tools to maximize the time spent with physicians.

Peer influence

Key opinion leaders

Key opinion leaders (KOL), or "thought leaders", are respected individuals, such as prominent medical school faculty, who influence physicians through their professional status. Pharmaceutical companies generally engage key opinion leaders early in the drug development process to provide advocacy and key marketing feedback. Some pharmaceutical companies identify key opinion leaders through direct inquiry of physicians (primary research). Recently, pharmaceutical companies have begun to use social network analysis to uncover thought leaders; because it does not introduce respondent bias, which is commonly found in primary research; it can identify and map out the entire scientific community for a disease state; and it has greater compliance with state and federal regulations; because physician prescribing patterns are not used to create the social network.

Alternatives to segmenting physicians purely on the basis of prescribing do exist, and marketers can call upon strategic partners who specialize in delineating which characteristics of true opinion leadership, a physician does or does not possess. Such analyses can help guide marketers in how to optimize KOL engagements as bona fide advisors to a brand, and can help shape clinical development and clinical data publication plans for instance, ultimately advancing patient care.

Colleagues

Physicians acquire information through informal contacts with their colleagues, including social events, professional affiliations, common hospital affiliations, and common medical school affiliations. Some pharmaceutical companies identify influential colleagues through commercially available prescription writing and patient level data. Doctor dinner meetings are an effective way for physicians to acquire educational information from respected peers. These meetings are sponsored by some pharmaceutical companies.

JOURNAL ARTICLES AND TECHNICAL DOCUMENTATION

Recent legal cases and US congressional hearings have provided access to pharmaceutical industry documents revealing new marketing strategies for drugs. Activities once considered independent of promotional intent, including continuing medical education and medical research, are used, including paying to publish articles about promoted drugs for the medical literature, and alleged suppression of unfavorable study results.

Private and Public Insurers

Evolution of marketing

The emergence of new media and technologies in recent years is quickly changing the pharmaceutical marketing landscape in the United States. Both physicians and users are increasing their reliance on the Internet as a source of health and medical information, prompting pharmaceutical marketers to look at digital channels for opportunities to reach their target audiences.

In 2008, 84% of U.S. physicians used the Internet and other technologies to access pharmaceutical, biotech or medical device information—a 20% increase from 2004. At the same time, sales reps are finding it more difficult to get time with doctors for in-person details. Pharmaceutical companies are exploring online marketing as an alternative way to reach physicians. Emerging e-promotional activities include live video detailing, online events, electronic sampling, and physician customer service portals such as PV Updates, MDLinx, Aptus Health (former Physicians Interactive), and Epocrates.

Direct-to-users marketers are also recognizing the need to shift to digital channels as audiences become more fragmented and the number of access points for news, entertainment and information multiplies. Standard television, radio and print direct-to-users (DTC) advertisements are less relevant than in the past, and companies are beginning to focus more on digital marketing efforts like product websites, online display advertising, search engine marketing, social media campaigns, place-based media and mobile advertising to reach the over 145 million U.S. adults online for health information.

In 2010, the FDA's Division of Drug Marketing, Advertising and Communications issued a warning letter concerning two unbranded consumer targeted Web sites sponsored by Novartis Pharmaceuticals Corporation as the websites promoted a drug for an unapproved use, the websites failed to disclose the risks associated with the use of the drug and made unsubstantiated dosing claims.

3

Product Decision and Strategies

Classification, product line and product mix decisions, product life cycle, product portfolio analysis; product positioning; New product decisions; Product branding, packaging and labelling decisions, and Product management in the pharmaceutical industry.

Decisions regarding the product, price, promotion and distribution channels are decisions on the elements of the "marketing mix". It can be argued that product decisions are probably the most crucial as the product is the very epitome of marketing planning. Errors in product decisions are legion.

These can include the imposition of a global standardised product where it is inapplicable, for example large horsepower tractors may be totally unsuitable for areas where small scale farming exists and where incomes are low; devolving decisions to affiliated countries which may let quality slip; and the attempt to sell products into a country without cognisance of cultural adaptation needs.

The decision whether to sell globally standardised or adapted products is too simplistic for today's market place. Many product decisions lie between these two extremes. Cognisance has also to be taken of the stage in the international life cycle, the organization's own product portfolio, its strengths and weaknesses and its global objectives.

Unfortunately, most developing, countries are in no position to compete on the world stage with many manufactured value-added products. Quality, or lack of it, is often the major letdown. Most developing countries are likely to be exporting raw materials or basic and high value agricultural produce for some time to come.

Product Planning is the ongoing process of identifying and articulating market requirements that define a product's feature set. Product planning serves as the basis for decisions about price, distribution and promotion. Product planning is the process of creating a product idea and following through on it until the product is introduced to the market. Additionally, a small company must have an exit strategy for its product in case the product does not sell. Product planning entails managing the product throughout its life using various marketing strategies, including product extensions or improvements, increased distribution, price changes and promotions.

Elements of Production Decisions

In decisions on producing or providing products and services in the international market it is essential that the production of the product or service is well planned and coordinated, both within and with other functional area of the firm, particularly marketing.

For example, in horticulture, it is essential that any supplier or any of his "out grower" (sub-contractor) can supply what he says he can. This is especially vital when contracts for supply are finalised, as failure to supply could incur large penalties. The main elements to consider are the production process itself, specifications, culture, the physical product, packaging, labelling, branding, warranty and service.

Production Process

The key question is, can we ensure continuity of supply? In manufactured products this may include decisions on the type of manufacturing process – artisanal, job, batch, flow line or group technology. However in many agricultural commodities factors like seasonality, perishability and supply and demand have to be taken into consideration.

Quantity and quality of horticultural crops are affected by a number of things. These include input supplies (or lack of them), finance and credit availability, variety (choice), sowing dates, product range and investment advice. Many of these items will be catered for in the contract of supply.

Specification

Specification is very important in agricultural products. Some markets will not take produce unless it is within their specification. Specifications are often set by the customer, but agents, standard authorities (like the EU or ITC Geneva) and trade associations can be useful sources.

Quality requirements often vary considerably. In the Middle East, red apples are preferred over green apples. In one example French red apples, well boxed, are sold at 55 dinars per box, whilst not so attractive Iranian greens are sold for 28 dinars per box. In export the quality standards are set by the importer. In Africa, Maritim (1991), found, generally, that there are no consistent standards for product quality and grading, making it difficult to do international trade regionally.

Culture

Product packaging, labeling, physical characteristics and marketing have to adapt to the cultural requirements when necessary. Religion, values, aesthetics, language and material culture all affect production decisions.

Again a number of these characteristics is governed by the customer or agent. For example, in beef products sold to the EU there are very strict quality requirements to be observed. In fish products, the Japanese demand more "exotic" types than, say, would be sold in the UK.

None of the dried fish products produced by the Zambians on Lake Kariba, and sold into the Lusaka market, would ever pass the hygiene laws if sold internationally. In sophisticated markets like seeds, the variety and range is so large that constant watch has to be kept on the new strains and varieties in order to be competitive.

Packaging

Packaging serves many purposes. It protects the product from damage which could be incurred in handling and transportation and also has a promotional aspect. It can be very expensive. Size, unit type, weight and volume are very important in packaging. For aircraft cargo the package needs to be light but strong, for sea cargo containers are often the best form.

The customer may also decide the best form of packaging. In horticultural produce, the developed countries often demand blister packs for mangetouts, beans, strawberries and so on, whilst for products like pineapples a sea container may suffice. Costs of packaging have always to be weighed against the advantage gained by it.

Increasingly, environmental aspects are coming into play. Packaging which is non-degradable plastic, for example is less in demanded. Bio-degradable, recyclable, reusable packaging is now the order of the day. This can be both expensive and demanding for many developing countries.

Labelling

Labelling not only serves to express the contents of the product, but may be promotional (symbols for example Cashel Valley Zimbabwe; HJ Heinz, Africafe, Tanzania). The EU is now putting very stringent regulations in force on labelling, even to the degree that the pesticides and insecticides used on horticultural produce have to be listed.

This could be very demanding for producers, especially small scale, ones where production techniques may not be standardised. Government labelling regulations vary from country to country. Bar codes are not widespread in Africa, but do assist in stock control.

Labels may have to be multilingual, especially if the product is a world brand. Translation could be a problem with many words being translated with difficulty. Again labelling is expensive, and in promotion terms non-standard labels are more expensive than standard ones. Requirements for crate labelling, etc. for international transportation will be dealt with later under documentation.

PHASES OF PRODUCT PLANNING

Developing the product concept

The first phase of product planning is developing the product concept. Marketing managers usually create ideas for new products by identifying certain problems that consumers face or various customers need. For example, a small computer retailer may see the need to create a computer repair division for the products it sells. After the product idea is conceived, managers will start planning the dimensions and features of the product. Some small companies will even develop a product mock-up or model.

Studying the Market

The next step in the product planning process is studying the competition. Secondary research usually provides details on key competitors and their market share, which is the percent of total sales that they hold in the marketplace. The business can then determine places in which it has an advantage over the competition to identify areas of opportunity. Market research is a complex task. It must include an analysis of products that are indirect competitors products manufactured by the company observed.

Market Research

A small company should consider doing both qualitative and quantitative marketing research for its new product. Focus groups are an example of qualitative information. Focus groups allow companies to ask their consumers about their likes and dislike of a product in small groups. A focus group allows the company to tweak the product concept before testing it through phone surveys—a more quantitative marketing research function. Phone surveys enables a company to test its product concept on a larger scale, the results of which are more predictable across the general population. Qualitative research is a method of inquiry employed in many different academic disciplines, traditionally in the social sciences, but also in market research and further contexts. Qualitative researchers aim to gather an in-depth understanding of human behavior and the reasons that govern such behavior. The qualitative method investigates the why and how of decision making, not just what, where, when. Hence, smaller but focused samples are more often used than large samples. Quantitative research refers to the systematic empirical investigation of social phenomena via statistical, mathematical or numerical data or computational techniques. The objective of quantitative research is to develop and employ mathematical models, theories and/or hypotheses pertaining to phenomena.

Market research is the one stage of product planning and it can be regarded as the way to accomplish the activity though designing questions, preparing the samples, collecting data and analyzing. It also can be considered as a kind of the communications between markets as research is always question-answer form.

For example, suppliers can collect buyers' suggestions and opinions through research and then get conclusion so that they can get buyers' satisfaction. In short, market research is applied to get market information, market segmentation, market trend and SWOT analysis such as consumer perceptions, market structure, distribution, past trends,strengths and weakness. The process to get these information can be divided into four parts which are definition, collection, analysis and interpretation. The steps are objectives, planning, data collection, data analysis, reporting and marketing decisions. Thereinto, data collection is the communication process as interviewers ask some questions and shoppers answer these and marketing decisions are results of communication.

Market researchers always use quantitative and qualitative research to differentiate the methods of investigation into those which are cared about getting an understanding of a subject and those which are involved in measuring things. At a word, quantitative and qualitative mean that one is based on quantity and the other one on quality. Qualitative research can be looked upon as a number of ways. Qualitative researchers do not need to interview so many people but they speak to really do count. The researchers are interested in asking 'How' questions not like 'how many'. Sampson(1967) has said that " it is centrally concerned with understanding things rather than with measuring them" this means that the lack of measurement can not make sure that the findings are accuracy. For example, the government has until recently used little qualitative research as it is worried that the public security would not believe these findings. Qualitative research is suited to solve the problem areas as following. The first one is basic market exploratory studies. For example, the research findings can be used to define consumer segmentations in relation to a product brand or understand the dimensions which differentiate between brands. The second one is new product development. For instance, product, packaging, positioning and advertising information can be collected through researching to confirm a new product proposition. The third one is diagnostic studies which is used to determine to what extent the brand image has changed since the start of an advertising campaign. (Gordon,Wendy,1943). The methods of qualitative research can be departed into observation and focus groups. Nowadays, observation is used wherever people think that watching is better to speaking and it plays an important role in researching people who can not articulate correctly and clearly what they think. It is frequently applied in shopping surveys particularly in-store, it regularly make customers try products and then ask them questions or do surveys. The results sometimes will be more reliable and creditable. Focus groups also can be called group discussions which is a tool on the basis of psychotherapy where it has found that if people are divided into small groups and asked to share their opinions and suggestions, they will be open up. Because there will generate a brainstorming effect in the groups so that a comment from one person can stimulate another one's ideas. Although qualitative research does not need many people to attend, one group is not enough that will cause the results are untypical. In general, there are always need four groups to cover a single respondent type. And the outcomes of group discussions are rely on the group leaders' abilities of structuring the discussion, conducting the meeting and analyzing and understanding the results.

Quantitative research is about understanding aspects of a market or what kinds of customers making up the market. And it can be split into soft and hard parts. Soft part means phenomena like customer attitudes and hard part is market size, brand shares and so on. Quantitative researchers are different from qualitative researchers, they pay more attention to asking 'What' questions. (Allen,Mike,1959) Quantitative research often provides three aims : description, forecasting and decision-making. (Franses,Philip Hans,1963) Quantitative market research means getting relevant information or measures from each single customer or shopper who are carrying out a census in the market. It is based on the strict sampling methods so that its data or results have levels of accuracy and can be taken to represent and stand for the population or to projecting. As the large basis will be collected in quantitative research, the types of quantitative data can be fallen into market measures, customer profiles or segmentation and attitudinal data. Firstly, market measures are used to quantify and describe a market like market size, the number of shares the suppliers or brands hold, how often does consumers purchase, schema of purchasing and so on. These data can help company or brand to plan or develop their product or marketing planning. Secondly, if a company want to plan a new product, it is necessary to know about the potential consumer base such as the age of people, what types of products or service they always use. There are various forms are included in profiling data like socio-demographics, geo-demographics customer behavior. The difference between market measures and consumer profiles is that only consumers can be the target people to collect profiling data. Thirdly, attitudinal data needs to collect the minds of individuals and then get results like awareness, beliefs, preference and so on. Attitude can influence behavior so that company or brand can use data to foresee customers' future behavior and then make product planning or business decision. On the other hand, there are many elements can change customers' attitude like price or appearance are changed. In a word, it is obvious that the communications between markets not only help each other to gain what they want but also develop the company or brand. It will make positive cycles between markets and then might promote the economy.

Thus, both of quantitative and qualitative research can be used to do market research to do the product planning and both of them are realized through communications so they can be regarded as kinds of communications between markets. The differences between quantitative and qualitative research can be summarized that qualitative research is always open-ended, more flexible, gives consumers more creativity, pays more attention to deeper understanding so that they can get deeper data and richer ideas and quantitative research are usually statistical and numerical measurement and people will be divided into groups to get sampling or comparisons.

Product Introduction

If the survey results prove favorable, the company may decide to sell the new product on a small scale or regional basis. During this time, the company will distribute the products in one or more cities. The company will run advertisements and sales promotions for the product, tracking sales results to determine the products potential success. If sales figures are favorable, the company will then expand distribution even further. Eventually, the company may be able to sell the product on a national basis.

Product Life Cycle

Product planning must also include managing the product through various stages of its product life cycle. These stages include the introduction, growth, maturity and decline stages. Sales are usually strong during the growth phase, while competition is low. However, continued success of the product will pique the interest of competitors, which will develop products of their own. The introduction of these competitive products may force a small company to lower its price. This low pricing strategy may help prevent the small company from losing market share. The company may also decide to better differentiate its product to keep its prices steady. For example, a small cell phone company may develop new, useful features on its cell phones that competitors do not have. PLC can be viewed as an important source of investment decision for the company.

If a company or brand wants to make sure that its products are successful, it needs to study the product life cycle to analyze market attractiveness and supplement the conclusion before it launches a new product or enters a new market. Product life cycle (PLC) theory is used to be explain the potential life cycle of a product from design to regression and the whole life cycle can be defined as four stages : introduction, growth, maturity and decline. Product life cycle plays an important role in marketing. The first reason is that the managers will follow the four stages to make product plans for pushing out new products. Secondly, the level and growth of sales will change a lot during the four stages so the managers need to adjust the product plan appropriately and timely. The last one is that the prices and costs will decrease markedly in the early stages of the product life cycle.

The first stage is introduction which means it is time for a company or brand to promote its new products. The goal of introduction is to attract customers' attention as much as possible and confirm the products' initial distribution, the company does not need to worry about the competition generally as the products are new. In this stage, there will have the first communication between marketers and customers as it will be the first time for consumers to know about the new products. In addition, the cost of the things will be high like research, testing and development and the sales are low as the new products' market is small.

The second stage is growth. In this stage, the new products have been accepted in the market and their sales and profits has begun to increase, the competition has happened so that the company will promote their quality to stay competitive. The products also have basic consumers' attention and can develop their loyal customers. There will have second communication as marketers can start to receive customers' feedback and then make improvements.

The third stage is maturity where the sales and profit have grown slowly and will reach their peak. The competitions between companies and brands will be fierce so that the companies will go out of their ways like providing higher quality products with a lower price or thinking about any improvements to survive in the competitions and make profits maximum.

The last one is decline which means the product is going to end and be discontinued. The sales of product will decrease until it is no longer in demand as it has become saturated, all the customers who want to buy this product has already got that. Then the company or brand will cut down the old products and pays attention to designing and developing the new products to gain back the customer base, stay in the markets and make profits.

In conclusion, although the differences will be happened if the product life cycle theory is applied to different types of products, it is important to the marketers. Product life cycle can show the strengths and weakness of a product so that the marketers can make a product successful and avoid loss through analyzing them. A good-managed product life cycle can also help a company or brand maximize the profit and stay in the markets for a long time. On the other hand, although the product life cycle theory seems that it just about products and marketers, it has the communications between marketers and customers. The interests, needs and feedback from the customers are necessary to the product life cycle. Because only the consumers have demand and they are interested in the new products, the products can start their introduction, and marketers need to collect and analyze the feedback and then adjust and improve their products to meet consumers' needs in order to increase the sales and profits in the growth and maturity stages.

New product Development

In business and engineering, new product development (NPD) covers the complete process of bringing a new product to market. A central aspect of NPD is product design, along with various business considerations. New product development is described broadly as the transformation of a market opportunity into a product available for sale. The product can be tangible (something physical which one can touch) or intangible (like a service, experience, or belief), though sometimes services and other processes are distinguished from "products." NPD requires an understanding of customer needs and wants, the competitive environment, and the nature of the market. Cost, time and quality are the main variables that drive customer needs. Aiming at these three variables, innovative companies develop continuous practices and strategies to better satisfy customer requirements and to increase their own market share by a regular development of new products. There are many uncertainties and challenges which companies must face throughout the process. The use of best practices and the elimination of barriers to communication are the main concerns for the management of the NPD .

Process Structure

The product development process typically consists of several activities that firms employ in the complex process of delivering new products to the market. A process managementapproach is used to provide a structure. Product development often overlaps much with the engineering design process, particularly if the new product being developed involves application of math and/or science. Every new product will pass through a series of stages/phases, including ideation among other aspects of design, as well as manufacturing and market introduction. In highly complex engineered products (e.g. aircraft, automotive, machinery), the NPD process can be likewise complex regarding management of personnel, milestones and deliverables. Such projects typically use an integrated product team approach. The process for managing large-scale complex engineering products is much slower (often 10-plus years) than that deployed for many types of consumer goods.

The product development process is articulated and broken down in many different ways, many of which often include the following phases/stages:

1. Fuzzy front-end (FFE) is the set of activities employed before the more formal and well defined requirements specification is completed. Requirements speak to wha-t th-e product should do or have, at varying degrees of specificity, in order to meet the perceived market or business need.
2. Product design is the development of both the high-level and detailed-level design of the product: which turns the what of the requirements into a specific how this particular product will meet those requirements. This typically has the most overlap with the engineering design process, but can also include industrial design and even purely aesthetic aspects of design. On the marketing and planning side, this phase ends at pre-commercialization analysis stage.
3. Product implementation often refers to later stages of detailed engineering design (e.g. refining mechanical or electrical hardware, or software, or goods or other product forms), as well as test process that may be used to validate that the prototype actually meets all design specifications that were established.
4. Fuzzy back-end or commercialization phase represent the action steps where the production and market launch occur.

The front-end marketing phases have been very well researched, with valuable models proposed. Peter Koen et al. provides a five-step front-end activity called front-end innovation: opportunity identification, opportunity analysis, idea genesis, idea selection, and idea and technology development. He also includes an engine in the middle of the five front-end stages and the possible outside barriers that can influence the process outcome. The engine represents the management driving the activities described. The front end of the innovation is the greatest area of weakness in the NPD process. This is mainly because the FFE is often chaotic, unpredictable and unstructured. Engineering design is the process whereby a technical solution is developed iteratively to solve a given problem The design stage is very important because at this stage most of the product life cycle costs are engaged. Previous research shows that 70–80% of the final product quality and 70% of the product entire life-cycle cost are determined in the product design phase, therefore the design-manufacturing interface represent the greatest opportunity for cost reduction. Design projects last from a few weeks to three years with an average of one year. Design and Commercialization phases usually start a very early collaboration. When the concept design is finished it will be sent to manufacturing plant for prototyping, developing a Concurrent Engineering approach by implementing practices such as QFD, DFM/DFA and more. The output of the design (engineering) is a set of product and process specifications – mostly in the form of drawings, and the output of manufacturing is the product ready for sale. Basically, the design team will develop drawings with technical specifications representing the future product, and will send it to the manufacturing plant to be executed. Solving product/process fit problems is of high priority in information communication design because 90% of the development effort must be scrapped if any changes are made after the release to manufacturing.

NPD Process

1. New Product Strategy – Innovators have clearly defined their goals and objectives for the new product.
2. Idea Generation – Collective brainstorming through internal and external sources.
3. Screening – Condense the number of brainstormed ideas.
4. Concept Testing – Structure an idea into a detailed concept.
5. Business Analysis – Understand the cost and profits of the new product and determining if they meet company objectives.
6. Product Development – Developing the product.
7. Market Testing – Marketing mix is tested through a trial run of the product.
8. Commercialization – Introducing the product to the public.

Models

Conceptual models have been designed in order to facilitate a smooth process. The concept adopted by IDEO, a successful design and consulting firm, is one of the most researched processes in regard to new product development and is a five-step procedure. These steps are listed in chronological order:

1. Understand and observe the market, the client, the technology, and the limitations of the problem;
2. Synthesize the information collected at the first step;
3. Visualise new customers using the product;
4. Prototype, evaluate and improve the concept;
5. Implementation of design changes which are associated with more technologically advanced procedures and therefore this step will require more time.

One of the first developed models that today companies still use in the NPD process is the Booz, Allen and Hamilton (BAH) Model, published in 1982. This is the best known model because it underlies the NPD systems that have been put forward later. This model represents the foundation of all the other models that have been developed afterwards. Significant work has been conducted in order to propose better models, but in fact these models can be easily linked to BAH model. The seven steps of BAH model are: new product strategy, idea generation, screening and evaluation, business analysis, development, testing, and commercialization.

A pioneer of NPD research in the consumers goods sector is Robert G. Cooper. Over the last two decades he conducted significant work in the area of NPD. The Stage-Gate model developed in the 1980s was proposed as a new tool for managing new products development processes. This was mainly applied to the consumers goods industry. The 2010 APQC benchmarking study reveals that 88% of U.S. businesses employ a stage-gate system to manage new products, from idea to launch. In return, the companies that adopt this system are reported to receive benefits such as improved teamwork, improved success rates, earlier detection of failure, a better launch, and even shorter cycle times – reduced by about 30%. These findings highlight the importance of the stage-gate model in the area of new product development.

Over the last few years, the Lean Startup movement has grown in popularity, challenging many of the assumptions inherent in the stage-gate model.

Marketing Considerations

There have been a number of approaches proposed for analyzing and responding to the marketing challenges of new product development. Two of these are the eight stagesprocess of Peter Koen of the Stevens Institute of Technology, and a process known as the fuzzy front end.

Fuzzy Front End

The Fuzzy Front End (FFE) is the messy "getting started" period of new product engineering development processes. It is also referred to as the "Front End of Innovation", or "Idea Management".

It is in the front end where the organization formulates a concept of the product to be developed and decides whether or not to invest resources in the further development of an idea. It is the phase between first consideration of an opportunity and when it is judged ready to enter the structured development process (Kim and Wilemon, 2007; Koen et al., 2001). It includes all activities from the search for new opportunities through the formation of a germ of an idea to the development of a precise concept. The Fuzzy Front End phase ends when an organization approves and begins formal development of the concept.

Although the Fuzzy Front End may not be an expensive part of product development, it can consume 50% of development time (see Chapter 3 of the Smith and Reinertsen reference below), and it is where major commitments are typically made involving time, money, and the product's nature, thus setting the course for the entire project and final end product. Consequently, this phase should be considered as an essential part of development rather than something that happens "before development," and its cycle time should be included in the total development cycle time.

Koen et al. (2001), distinguish five different front-end elements (not necessarily in a particular order):

1. Opportunity Identification
2. Opportunity Analysis
3. Idea Genesis
4. Idea Selection
5. Idea and Technology Development

- The first element is the opportunity identification. In this element, large or incremental business and technological chances are identified in a more or less structured way. Using the guidelines established here, resources will eventually be allocated to new projects.... which then lead to a structured NPPD (New Product & Process Development) strategy.
- The second element is the opportunity analysis. It is done to translate the identified opportunities into implications for the business and technology specific context of the company. Here extensive efforts may be made to align ideas to target customer groups and do market studies and/or technical trials and research.
- The third element is the idea genesis, which is described as evolutionary and iterative process progressing from birth to maturation of the opportunity into a tangible idea. The process of the idea genesis can be made internally or come from outside inputs, e.g. a supplier offering a new material/technology or from a customer with an unusual request.
- The fourth element is the idea selection. Its purpose is to choose whether to pursue an idea by analyzing its potential business value.
- The fifth element is the idea and technology development. During this part of the front-end, the business case is developed based on estimates of the

total available market, customer needs, investment requirements, competition analysis and project uncertainty. Some organizations consider this to be the first stage of the NPPD process (i.e., Stage 0).

A universally acceptable definition for Fuzzy Front End or a dominant framework has not been developed so far. In a glossary of PDMA, it is mentioned that the Fuzzy Front End generally consists of three tasks: strategic planning, idea generation, and pre-technical evaluation. These activities are often chaotic, unpredictable, and unstructured. In comparison, the subsequent new product development process is typically structured, predictable, and formal. The term Fuzzy Front End was first popularized by Smith and Reinertsen (1991). R.G. Cooper (1988) it describes the early stages of NPPD as a four-step process in which ideas are generated (I), subjected to a preliminary technical and market assessment (II) and merged to coherent product concepts (III) which are finally judged for their fit with existing product strategies and portfolios (IV).

The Phase Zero of the Stage-Gate Model of New Product Development

The Stage-Gate model of NPD predevelopment activities are summarised in Phase zero and one, in respect to earlier definition of predevelopment activities:

1. Preliminary
2. Technical assessment
3. Source-of-supply assessment: suppliers and partners or alliances
4. Market research: market size and segmentation analysis, VoC (voice of the customer) research
5. Product idea testing
6. Customer value assessment
7. Product definition
8. Business and financial analysis

These activities yield essential information to make a Go/No-Go to Development decision. These decisions represent the Gates in the Stage-Gate model.

EARLY PHASE OF THE INNOVATION PROCESS

A conceptual model of Front-End Process was proposed which includes early phases of the innovation process. This model is structured in three phases and three gates:

- Phase 1: Environmental screening or opportunity identification stage in which external changes will be analysed and translated into potential business opportunities.
- Phase 2: Preliminary definition of an idea or concept.
- Phase 3: Detailed product, project or service definition, and Business planning.

The gates are:

- Opportunity screening
- Idea evaluation
- Go/No-Go for development

The final gate leads to a dedicated new product development project. Many professionals and academics consider that the general features of Fuzzy Front End (fuzziness, ambiguity, and uncertainty) make it difficult to see the FFE as a structured process, but rather as a set of interdependent activities (e.g. Kim and Wilemon, 2002). However, Husig et al., 2005 argue that front-end not need to be fuzzy, but can be handled in a structured manner. In fact Carbone showed that when using the front end success factors in an integrated process, product success is increased. Peter Koen argues that in the FFE for incremental, platform and radical projects, three separate strategies and processes are typically involved. The traditional Stage Gate (TM) process was designed for incremental product development, namely for a single product. The FFE for developing a new platform must start out with a strategic vision of where the company wants to develop products and this will lead to a family of products. Projects for breakthrough products start out with a similar strategic vision, but are associated with technologies which require new discoveries.

Activity view on Fuzzy-Front End

Predevelopment is the initial stage in NPD and consists of numerous activities, such as:

- product strategy formulation and communication
- opportunity identification and assessment
- idea generation
- product definition
- project planning
- executive reviews

Economical analysis, benchmarking of competitive products and modeling and prototyping are also important activities during the front-end activities.

The outcomes of FFE are the:

- mission statement
- customer needs
- details of the selected idea
- product definition and specifications
- economic analysis of the product
- the development schedule
- project staffing and the budget

- a business plan aligned with corporate strategy

Incremental, platform and breakthrough products include:

- Incremental products are considered to be cost reductions, improvements to existing product lines, additions to existing platforms and repositioning of existing products introduced in markets.
- Breakthrough products are new to the company or new to the world and offer a 5–10 times or greater improvement in performance combined with a 30–50% or greater reduction in costs.
- Platform products establish a basic architecture for a next generation product or process and are substantially larger in scope and resources than incremental projects.

Strategies

- Lean product development
- Design for six sigma
- Quality function deployment
- Phase–gate model
- User-centered design

Management

Companies must take a holistic approach to managing this process and must continue to innovate and develop new products if they want to grow and prosper.

- CUSTOMER CENTERED New Product Development. Focuses on:
- Finding new ways to solve customer problems.
- Create more customer-satisfying experience

Companies often rely on technology, but the real success comes from understanding customer needs and values.

The most successful companies were the ones that:

- Differentiated from others
- Solved major customer problems
- Offered a compelling customer value proposition
- Engaged customer directly
- TEAM BASED New Product Development
- An approach:
- To deserving new products in which various company's departments work closely together overlapping the steps in the product development process in order to:

- Save time
- Increase effectiveness
- Company departments work closely together in cross functional teams overlapping the steps in the product development process (to save time and increase effectiveness).
- Those departments are: legal, marketing, finances, design and manufacturing, suppliers and customer companies.
- If there is a problem, all the company can work.
- SYSTEMATIC New Product Development
- Development process should be holistic (alternative) and systematic not to good ideas die.
- This process is installed on Innovation Management System that collect, review, evaluate new product ideas and manage
- the company appoints to a senior person to be the Innovation Manager who encourage all the company
- employees, suppliers, distributors and dealers to become involved in finding and developing new products.
- Then, there is a Cross-Functional Innovation Management Committee which:
- Evaluate new products ideas
- Help bringing good ideas
- To sum up, New-Product success requires:
- New ways to create valued customer experience, from generating and screening new product ideas to create and roll out want-satisfying products.
- New Product Development IN TURBULENT TIMES
- When we are in a tough economic situation usually management reduces spending on: new-product development. Usually it is done from a short-sighted point of view.
- Tough times might even call for:
- Greater new-product development, offering solutions for changing customer needs and tastes.
- Innovation helps
- Making the company more competitive
- Positioning it better for future.
- Virtual product development
- Uses collaboration technology to remove need for co-located teams
- Reduces G&A overhead costs of consulting firms

- Advent of 24-hour development cycle

Related Fields

- End user
- Brand management
- Engineering
- Industrial design
- Marketing
- Product management

Promotion (marketing)

In marketing, promotion refers to any type of marketing communication used to inform or persuade target audiences of the relative merits of a product, service, brand or issue. The aim of promotion is to increase awareness, create interest, generate sales or create brand loyalty. It is one of the basic elements of the market mix, which includes the four P's ,i.e., Product, Price, Place, Promotion.

Promotion is also one of the elements in the promotional mix or promotional plan. These are personal selling, advertising, sales promotion, direct marketing publicity and may also include event marketing, exhibitions and trade shows. A promotional plan specifies how much attention to pay to each of the elements in the promotional mix, and what proportion of the budget should be allocated to each element.

Promotion covers the methods of communication that a marketer uses to provide information about its product. Information can be both verbal and visual.

Etymology and Usage

The term, "promotion' derives from the Old French, promocion meaning to "move forward", "push onward" or to "advance in rank or position" which in turn, comes from the Latin, promotionem meaning "a moving forward". The word entered the English language in the 14th century.

The use of the term promotion to refer to "advertising or publicity" is very modern and is first recorded in 1925. It may be a contraction of a related term, sales promotion, which is one element in the larger set of tools used in marketing communications. The terms, promotion and marketing communications can be used synonymously, but in practice, the latter is more widely used.

Purpose

There are three objectives of promotion. These are:

1. To present information to consumers and others.
2. To increase demand.
3. To differentiate a product.

The purpose of a promotion and thus its promotional plan can have a wide range, including: sales increases, new product acceptance, creation of brand equity, positioning, competitive retaliations, or creation of a corporate image.

The term 'promotion' tends to be used internally by the marketing function. To the public or the market, phrases like "special offer" are more common. Examples of a fully integrated, long-term, and large-scale promotion are My Coke Rewards in the USA or Coke Zone in the UK and Pepsi Stuff.

Types

There have been different ways to promote a product in person or with different media. Both person and media can be either physically real or virtual/electronic.

In a Physical Environment

Promotions can be held in physical environments at special events such as concerts, festivals, trade shows, and in the field, such as in grocery or department stores. Interactions in the field allow immediate purchases. The purchase of a product can be incentive with discounts (i.e., coupons), free items, or a contest. This method is used to increase the sales of a given product. Interactions between the brand and the customer are performed by a brand ambassador or promotional model who represents the product in physical environments. Brand ambassadors or promotional models are hired by a marketing company, which in turn is booked by the brand to represent the product or service. Person-to-person interaction, as opposed to media-to-person involvement, establishes connections that add another dimension to promotion. Building a community through promoting goods and services can lead to brand loyalty.

Traditional Media

Examples of traditional media include print media such as newspapers and magazines, electronic media such as radio and television, and outdoor media such as banner or billboardadvertisements. Each of these platforms provide ways for brands to reach consumers with advertisements.

Digital Media

Digital media, which includes Internet, social networking and social media sites, is a modern way for brands to interact with consumers as it releases news, information and advertising from the technological limits of print and broadcast infrastructures. Digital media is currently the most effective way for brands to reach their consumers on a daily basis. Over 2.7 billion people are online globally, which is about 40% of the world's population. 67% of all Internet users globally use social media.

Mass communication has led to modern marketing strategies to continue focusing on brand awareness, large distributions and heavy promotions. The fast-paced environment of digital media presents new methods for promotion to utilize new tools now available through technology. With the rise of technological advances, promotions can be done outside of local contexts and across geographic borders to reach a greater number of potential consumers. The goal of a promotion is then to reach the most people possible in a time efficient and a cost efficient manner.

Social media, as a modern marketing tool, offers opportunities to reach larger audiences in an interactive way. These interactions allow for conversation rather than simply educating the customer. Facebook, Snapchat, Instagram, Twitter, Pinterest, Google Plus, Tumblr, as well as alternate audio and media sites like SoundCloud and Mixcloud allow users to interact and promote music online with little to no cost. You can purchase and buy ad space as well as potential customer interactions stores as Likes, Followers, and clicks to your page with the use of third parties. As a participatory media culture, social media platforms or social networking sites are forms of mass communication that, through media technologies, allow large amounts of product and distribution of content to reach the largest audience possible. However, there are downsides to virtual promotions as servers, systems, and websites may crash, fail, or become overloaded with information. You also can stand risk of losing uploaded information and storage and at a use can also be effected by a number of outside variables.

Brands can explore different strategies to keep consumers engaged. One popular tool is branded entertainment, or creating some sort of social game for the user. The benefits of such a platform include submersing the user in the brand's content. Users will be more likely to absorb and not grow tired of advertisements if they are, for example, embedded in the game as opposed to a bothersome pop-up ad.

Personalizing advertisements is another strategy that can work well for brands, as it can increase the likelihood that the brand will be anthropomorphized by the consumer. Personalization increases click-through intentions when data has been collected about the consumer.

Brands must navigate the line between effectively promoting their content to consumers on social media and becoming too invasive in consumers' lives. Vivid Internet ads that include devices such as animation might increase a user's initial attention to the ad. However, this may be seen as a distraction to the user if they are trying to absorb a different part of the site such as reading text. Additionally, when brands make the effort of overtly collecting data about their consumers and then personalizing their ads to them, the consumer's relationship with the advertisements, following this data collection, is frequently positive. However, when data is covertly collected, consumers can quickly feel like the company betrayed their trust. It is important for brands to utilize personalization in their ads, without making the consumer feel vulnerable or that their privacy has been betrayed.

4

Qualitative and Quantitative Marketing Research in Pharma Marketing

Today's competitive arena in pharma marketing and business demands tapping into the psyche of consumers, physicians, and everyone in between, including family members and medical professionals. While the debate of qualitative vs. quantitative research and which one is superior is a long-winded one, the challenge in the current world of marketing is to blend the two in order to gain actionable results in reaching these crucial groups of people.

The Crucial Market Research

Leading pharma companies recognize the importance of market research, which includes competitive intelligence, customer insights, product positioning, and behavioral trends. They are aware that they must understand patient and physician behaviors, perspectives, and attitudes in order to successfully and effectively position new products in the market.

While it's true that there are several types of methods used to gain quantitative market information, a mainstay for qualitative input is the focus group. Is your pharmaceutical company getting all you can from your focus group research efforts?

Specialists believe that pharma can realize value that goes beyond the primary objectives of research and gain better insight and data by identifying more targeted objectives, using improved technologies, and developing better designed studies overall.

Focus Groups and Pharma Marketing

One of the main reasons focus groups are used is to determine the practices, attitudes, and knowledge of those who are participating. These groups are also an effective way to obtain guidance on clinical trials, test promotional elements, and make decisions for products.

However, experts advise that focus groups do provide valuable information – but the results are qualitative, and not quantitative. This is one common mistake made by pharma companies today.

"Focus groups shouldn't be used for quantitative measurement," Dr. Vanderveer, Ph.D., CEO of V2 Inc., says. "The unit of analysis when 10 doctors are together is really the group. It doesn't make sense to say 6 out of 10 doctors in the group said `x.' Because physicians play off each other, we don't get a pure read of the knowledge, attitudes, and practices of any one physician in the group."

"The rest is generally spent on quantitative types of market research, ranging from the use of the Internet to conducting surveys, tracking studies, modeling discrete choice studies, and using statistical metrics," he says.

Furthermore, some companies run focus groups that are quasi quantitative in nature, says Ken Berwitz, President of Ken Berwitz Marketing Research and the National Qualitative Centers, Inc. "Clients have the moderator ask one question, get an answer from everybody, and then ask the next question, with no probing, interaction, or synergy from members of the group," he says. "This really isn't a focus group. The purpose of the focus group is not to come to conclusions; at least it shouldn't be. The purpose should be to get ideas and direction, which are then tested quantitatively in a statistically viable way."

OTHER COMMON MISTAKES PHARMA MARKETERS MAKE

Another mistake commonly made by companies is that they use results as the only vehicle for making decisions. Instead, they should use research as "fodder' for marketing decisions. Phil Deschamps, President of Gerbig, Snell/Weisheimer says, "Human nature is to rely on objective metrics to make decisions. The lure of being able to say `market research said so' is a shield. Market research should be used as a sword to help us make better marketing decisions."

Ron Brand, group director of salesforce effectiveness consulting at IMS Health agrees: "Primary research is important, but it shouldn't be used in isolation," he says. "There is additional information that can be brought to bear for segmentation purposes. To extract greater value, marketers have to link those primary variables with a physician's demographics and behaviors in terms of prescribing patterns and with other influences such as managed care. Combining all of these elements presents a more complete and actionable picture."

Select the Right Methods

One of the first decisions companies must make when it comes to market research is to select the right methodology for its objectives, whether it be a survey, interviews, focus groups, or online sessions. Start by taking into account all the business decisions that require third party input, then decide how to best gain meaningful data. Focus groups should be used to obtain knowledge that extends farther than the objectives of a particular research project.

Regardless of the methodology chosen, pharma marketers must make sure that personal bias doesn't skew results – this is especially true in a focus group setting, since interpretation of results is subjective. To guard against bias, more than one person should interpret the results.

In addition to the need to be careful when interpreting information is the need for a well-controlled environment.

Justina Lambert, VP of marketing at SigmaTau Pharmaceuticals Inc. explains, "Du ing focus-group sessions, often there are people who have very strong opinions or personalities and naturally that person begins to influence the opinions of the other participants. During one focus group, we had a participant who was very outspoken about our product and had a negative perception about dialysis patients in general. After a very short period of time, we started to see the other focus group participants clam up or follow the lead of this outspoken person rather than presenting their own opinions and ideas. That skews the entire focus group. But by using backup survey data we can ensure the results of a focus group are valid."

Improve Your Marketing Process

Today, the best way to get the most from your pharma company's market research budget is to invest the resources and time needed for proper implementation. Proper planning is crucial to yield the best results. Oftentimes, pharma groups look for the easiest, quickest, and cheapest approach for research, but it isn't always the best way. Technology is the key to interpreting data and gaining insights from collected information. This will help reveal to upper management what the "real world is like" by assembling a presentation of realistic interviews.

Physicians and Pharma Marketing

An effective way to obtain that "real world" outlook is to get doctors out of "doctor mode." According to Deschamps, "The methodology of the focus group, the ability of the moderator, and the questions should be structured to remove doctors from their analytical comfort zone," he says. "Doctors are trained to look unemotionally at situations and to come up with the best logical and left-brain approach to treat their patients. In the context of a focus group, where more often than not a company is trying to determine product positioning or marketing concepts, it is important to have the physician become a consumer."

He goes on to explain that the manner in which physicians answer questions also leads to vital information. "When the moderator asks, 'how would you diagnose a particular patient?' or 'what's going through your mind?', it takes physicians back to their comfort zone and we lose the opportunity to have them provide a sincere, honest reaction because these are questions they answer many times in the course of a day. Someone listening in on a focus group we may hear a lot of conversation, but we're really not learning anything new. By taking physicians out of their comfort zone and asking the right questions, we can tap into their emotions. Such as, `what emotion do you have when you see a patient with a certain disease?' Or, `how did you feel when you were able to satisfactorily treat the patient?' By getting physicians to open up emotionally, focus groups give marketers some insight into their psyche and provide information that we can capitalize on."

THE TRAP OF DOING TOO MUCH WITH TOO LITTLE TIME

Companies must remain realistic with their expectations; questions that will be asked need to be carefully and thoughtfully designed. The moderator has to be well-versed and experienced in orchestrating the flow of discussions, maintaining the right timing, and asking the right questions at the best opportunities.

"Often clients add too many components and the outcome is a history of pharmaceuticals part one," Mr. Berwitz says. "When that happens, the moderator is forced to cut off rich discussions, which would have yielded important information, in order to cover everything on the agenda. Companies need to prioritize and identify the most important elements to be addressed. Instead of having 10 issues up for discussion, cut the number down to six. Unless those critical issues are identified and there is enough time to fully explore them, all the richness of the focus group is lost. Focus groups can't be treated as economy centers."

The questions that the moderator is asking are vital to ensure that the company is getting the exact information that it is looking for," Ms. Lambert says. "Often companies have a list of questions, then leave them in the hands of the individuals or the group who is conducting the focus group. Naturally at the end of the process, the company may very well not get what it is looking for."

Qualitative Marketing Research

Qualitative marketing research involves a natural or observational examination of the philosophies that govern consumer behavior. The direction and framework of the research is often revised as new information is gained, allowing the researcher to evaluate issues and subjects in an in-depth manner. The quality of the research produced is heavily dependent on the skills of the researcher and is influenced by researcher bias.

Data Collection

Qualitative marketing researchers collect data ranging from focus group, case study, participation observation, innovation game and individual depth interview.

Focus group

The focus group is marketing research technique for qualitative data that involves a small group of people (6–10) that share a common set characteristics (demographics, attitudes, etc.) and participate in a discussion of predetermined topics led by a moderator. There are opportunities to conduct focus groups with the use of focus group software. There are many types of focus group as well, but they always involve discussion among the group(s). The problem of the focus group is the issue of observer dependency: the results obtained are influenced by the researcher or his own reading of the group's discussion, raising questions of validity. Non-verbal cues, which may contradict the views participants articulate, are important and can easily be missed if the researcher is not familiar with visual cues, body language and other non verbal cues.

Qualitative Case study

Qualitative case study methodology provides tools for researchers to study complex phenomena within their contexts. Because it only studies one case, so it is very up-close, in-depth. It contains high levels of internal validity (the extent to which one is able to say that no other variables except the one being studied caused the result), but the external validityis low. Customer behaviour is a good example for qualitative market research.

Participation observation

Participation observation is watching participants' behavior in real world settings without trying to manipulate their actions. This method is high in external validity but low in internal validity.

Innovation game

Innovation game refers to a form of primary market research developed by Luke Hohmann where customers play a set of directed games as a means of generating feedback about a product or service. A facilitator explains the game(s) to be played and controls the paces, monitors the participants' levels and manages the time. There are many types of innovation games, such as 20/20 vision, me and my shadow, and buy a feature.

Individual Depth Interviews

In-depth interviews, also called IDIs, have been an integral component of market research since its inception in the 1920s. This method is useful when you want detailed information about a person's thoughts and behaviors or want to explore new issues in depth. One can get unique points from each respondent, and their answers will not be influenced by other people as in a focus group. In-depth interviews are held one-on-one between the respondent and the interview via a telephone, conducted in person, or through an online platform (increasingly common).

The primary advantage of in-depth interviews is the amount of detailed information provided as compared to other data collection methods, such as surveys.

Another advantage is reaching respondents that are geographically dispersed, which cannot occur in a focus group. This method is often used to refine future research or provide context to future studies. The primary disadvantage of in-depth interviews is the time to conduct, transcribe, and analyze. As such, this method could have higher costs associated with it than other methods.

Uses

Qualitative market research is often part of survey methodology, including telephone surveys and consumer satisfaction surveys. We apply the qualitative market research when:

- New product idea generation and development
- Investigating current or potential product/service/brand positioning and marketing strategy
- Strengths and weaknesses of products/brands
- Understanding dynamics of purchase decision dynamics
- Studying reactions to advertising and public relations campaigns, other marketing communications, graphic identity/branding, package design, etc.
- Exploring market segments, such as demographic and customer groups
- Assessing the usability of websites or other interactive products or services
- Understanding perceptions of a company, brand, category and product

Typical General Procedure

1. Setting the question
2. Deciding the objectives
3. Planning research design
4. Select data collection techniques
5. Sample design
6. Data collection
7. Analysis
8. Do the report

Advantages

- More detailed and in-depth questions
- Reduced cost, since the scale of this kind of research is small

- Discovering the "why" behind certain behaviors
- Quick turnaround: the direction of the research can be changed easily

Disadvantages

- Issues on confidentiality and anonymity can pose problems during presentation of findings.
- If researcher does not have enough skills such as communication skill, the quality of research is likely to be low.
- The sample size is relatively small, the result may not be very accurate.
- Qualitative research produces large amounts of data which requires a tremendous amount of work and labor on the part of the researcher.

Vs. Quantitative Marketing Research

Objective

Qualitative research is usually aimed to have an inside look about opinions or motivations, while quantitative research uses data to simplify the result.

Sample

Qualitative research usually has a smaller sample size than quantitative research due to the complexity of its data.

Data collection

Qualitative research usually uses unstructured or semi-structured techniques to collect data, e.g. individual depth interviews or group discussions, while quantitative research only uses structured techniques such as online questionnaires, on-street or telephone interviews.

Outcom

The outcomes of qualitative marketing research are usually conclusive and cannot be used to make generalizations about the population of interest, instead developing an initial understanding and sound base for further decision making. The findings of quantitative marketing research are conclusive and usually descriptive in nature.

Data analysis

Coding

Coding is an interpretive technique that both organizes the data and provides a means to introduce the interpretations of it into certain quantitative methods.

Qualitative research is a scientific method of observation to gather non-numerical data. This type of research "refers to the meanings, concepts definitions, characteristics, metaphors, symbols, and description of things" and not to their "counts or measures. This research answers how and when a certain phenomenon occurs." Qualitative research approaches are employed across many academic disciplines, focusing particularly on the human elements of the social and natural sciences; in less academic contexts, areas of application include qualitative market research, business, service demonstrations by non-profits, and journalism.

As a field of study, qualitative approaches include research concepts and methods from multiple established academic fields. The aim of a qualitative research project may vary with the disciplinary background, such as a psychologist seeking in-depth understanding of human behavior and the reasons that govern such behavior for example. Qualitative methods are best for researching many of the whyand how questions of human experience, in making a decision for example (not just what, where, when, or "who"); and have a strong basis in the field of sociology to understand government and social programs. Qualitative research is widely used by political science, social work, and education researchers.

In the conventional view of statisticians, qualitative methods produce explanations only of the particular cases studied (e.g., as part of an ethnography of a newly implemented government program), any general conclusions beyond the study context are considered tentative propositions (informed assertions), since the general propositions are not usually arrived at on the basis of statistical theory. Quantitative methods are therefore needed, to seek mathematical evidence and justification for such hypotheses for further research.

In contrast, a qualitative researcher might argue that understanding of a phenomenon or situation or event, comes from exploring the totality of the situation (e.g., phenomenology, symbolic interactionism), often with access to large amounts of "hard data" of a nonnumerical form. It may begin as a grounded theory approach with the researcher having no previous understanding of the phenomenon; or the study may commence with propositions and proceed in a 'scientific and empirical way' throughout the research process (e.g., Bogdan & Taylor, 1990).

"We can distinguish between those which follow the logic of quantitative methods in their rules and criteria and make generalizations in a numerical sense (i. e. from numerous cases to more numerous cases), and those clearly qualitative methods where interpretations and generalizations are not based on the frequency of occurrence of certain social phenomena but on a logic of generalizing from an individual case, whether this case is a personal biography, an organization or a particular milieu or social setting; this includes making microscopic and thick descriptions (see Geertz 1973) of the phenomena in which we are interested, likewise with the aim of generalizing from an individual case."

—Gabriele Rosenthal, (2018: 13): Interpretive Social Research. An Introduction. Göttingen: Universitätsverlag Göttingen.

A popular method of qualitative research is the case study (Stake 1995, Yin 1989), which examines in depth 'purposive samples' to better understand a phenomenon (e.g., support to families; Racino, 1999); the case study method exemplifies the qualitative researchers' preference for depth, detail, and context, often working with smaller and more focused samples, compared with the large samples of primary interest to statistical researchers seeking general laws.

Qualitative methods are an integral component of the five angles of analysis fostered by the data percolation methodology. These methods may be used alongside quantitative methods, scholarly or lay reviews of the literature, interviews with experts, and computer simulation, as part of multimethod attitude to data collection and analysis (called Triangulation).

To help navigate the heterogeneous landscape of qualitative research, one can further think of qualitative inquiry in terms of 'means' and 'orientation'. In particular, one could argue that qualitative researchers often reject natural science models of truth, prefer inductive, hypothesis-generating research processes and procedures (over hypothesis-testing models), are oriented towards investigations of meaning(s) rather than behaviour, and prefer data in the form of words and images, that are ideally naturally derived (e.g. in-depth observation as opposed to experimentation).History

Sociologist Earl Babbie notes that qualitative research is "at once very old and very new." He documents that qualitative methods have been used for several centuries, but anthropologists brought qualitative field research methods to the forefront through their 19th century observations of preliterate societies.

Robert Bogdan in his advanced courses on qualitative research traces the history of the development of the fields, and their particular relevance to disability and including the work of his colleague Robert Edgerton and a founder of participant observation, Howard S. Becker. As Robert Bogdan and Sari Biklen describe in their education text, "historians of qualitative research have never, for instance, included Freud or Piaget as developers of the qualitative approach, yet both relied on case studies, observations and indepth interviewing".

In the early 1900s, some researchers rejected positivism, the theoretical idea that there is an objective world which we can gather data from and "verify" this data through empiricism. These researchers embraced a qualitative research paradigm, attempting to make qualitative research as "rigorous" as quantitative research and creating myriad methods for qualitative research. Such developments were necessary as qualitative researchers won national center awards, in collaboration with their research colleagues at other universities and departments; and university administrations funded Ph.D.s in both arcnas through the ensuing decades. Most theoretical constructs involve a process of qualitative analysis and understanding, and construction of these concepts (e.g., Wolfensberger's social role valorization theories).

In the 1970s and 1980s, the increasing ubiquity of computers aided in qualitative analyses, several journals with a qualitative focus emerged, and postpositivism gained recognition in the academy. In the late 1980s, questions of identity emerged, including issues of race, class, gender, and discourse communities, leading to research and writing becoming more reflexive. Throughout the 1990s, the concept of a passive observer/researcher was rejected, and qualitative research became more participatory and activist-oriented with support from the federal branches, such as the National Institute on Disability Research and Rehabilitation (NIDRR) of the US Department of Education (e.g., Rehabilitation Research and Training Centers for Family and Community Living, 1990). Also, during this time, researchers began to use mixed-method approaches, indicating a shift in thinking of qualitative and quantitative methods as intrinsically incompatible. However, this history is not apolitical, as this has ushered in a politics of "evidence" (e.g., evidence-based practices in health and human services) and what can count as "scientific" research in scholarship, a current, ongoing debate in the academy.

DATA COLLECTION, ANALYSIS AND FIELD RESEARCH DESIGN

Qualitative researchers face many choices for techniques to generate data ranging from grounded theory development and practice, narratology, storytelling, transcript poetry, biographical narrative interviews, classical ethnography, state or governmental studies, research and service demonstrations, focus groups, case studies, participant observation, qualitative review of statistics in order to predict future happenings, or shadowing, among many others. Qualitative methods are used in various methodological approaches, such as action research which has sociological basis, or actor-network theory.

The interview (structured, semi-structured or unstructured) is a common source of data on the qualities/categories of interest. Other sources include focus groups, observation (without a predefined theory like statistical theory in mind for example), reflective field notes, texts, pictures, photographs and other images, interactions and practice captured on audio or video recordings, public (e.g. official) personal documents, historical items, and websites and social media.

To analyse qualitative data, the researcher seeks meaning from all of the data that is available. The data may be categorized and sorted into patterns (i.e., pattern or thematic analyses) as the primary basis for organizing and reporting the study findings (e.g., activities in the home; interactions with government). Qualitative researchers, often associated with the education field, typically rely on the following methods for gathering information: Participant Observation, Non-participant Observation, Field Notes, Reflexive Journals, Biographical Narrative Interviews, Structured Interview, Semi-structured Interview, Unstructured Interview, and Analysis of documents and materials.

The ways of participating and observing can vary widely from setting to setting as exemplified by Helen Schwartzman's primer on Ethnography in Organizations

(1993). or Anne Copeland and Kathleen White's "Studying Families" (1991). Participant observation is a strategy of reflexive learning, not a single method of observing. and has been described as a continuum of between participation and observation. In participant observation researchers typically become members of a culture, group, or setting, and adopt roles to conform to that setting. In doing so, the aim is for the researcher to gain a closer insight into the culture's practices, motivations, and emotions. It is argued that the researchers' ability to understand the experiences of the culture may be inhibited if they observe without participating.

The data that is obtained is streamlined (texts of thousands of pages in length) to a definite theme or pattern, or representation of a theory or systemic issue or approach. This step in a theoretical analysis or data analytic technique is further worked on (e.g., gender analysis may be conducted; comparative policy analysis may be developed). An alternative research hypothesis is generated which finally provides the basis of the research statement for continuing work in the fields.

Some distinctive qualitative methods are the use of focus groups and key informant interviews, the latter often identified through sophisticated and sometimes, elitist, snowballing techniques. The focus group technique (e.g., Morgan, 1988) involves a moderator facilitating a small group discussion between selected individuals on a particular topic, with video and handscribed data recorded, and is useful in a coordinated research approach studying phenomenon in diverse ways in different environments with distinct stakeholders often excluded from traditional processes. This method is a particularly popular in market research and testing new initiatives with users/workers.

The research then must be "written up" into a report, book chapter, journal paper, thesis or dissertation, using descriptions, quotes from participants, charts and tables to demonstrate the trustworthiness of the study findings.

In qualitative research, the idea of recursivity is expressed in terms of the nature of its research procedures, which may be contrasted with experimental forms of research design. From the experimental perspective, its major stages of research (data collection, data analysis, discussion of the data in context of the literature, and drawing conclusions) should be each undertaken once (or at most a small number of times) in a research study. In qualitative research however, all of the four stages above may be undertaken repeatedly until one or more specific stopping conditions are met, reflecting a nonstatic attitude to the planning and design of research activities. An example of this dynamicism might be when the qualitative researcher unexpectedly changes their research focus or design midway through a research study, based on their 1st interim data analysis, and then makes further unplanned changes again based on a 2nd interim data analysis; this would be a terrible thing to do from the perspective of an (predefined) experimental study of the same thing. Qualitative researchers would argue that their recursivity in developing the relevant evidence and reasoning, enables the researcher to be more open to unexpected results, more open to the potential of building new constructs, and the possibility of integrating them with the explanations developed continuously throughout a study.

Specialized uses of Qualitative Research

Qualitative methods are often part of survey methodology, including telephone surveys and consumer satisfaction surveys.

In fields that study households, a much debated topic is whether interviews should be conducted individually or collectively (e.g. as couple interviews).

One traditional and specialized form of qualitative research is called cognitive testing or pilot testing which is used in the development of quantitative survey items. Survey items are piloted on study participants to test the reliability and validity of the items. This approach is similar to psychological testing using an intelligence test like the WAIS (Wechsler Adult Intelligence Survey) in which the interviewer records "qualitative" (i.e., clinical observations)throughout the testing process. Qualitative research is often useful in a sociological lens. Although often ignored, qualitative research is of great value to sociological studies that can shed light on the intricacies in the functionality of society and human interaction.

There are several different research approaches, or research designs, that qualitative researchers use. In the academic social sciences, the most frequently used qualitative research approaches include the following points:

1. Basic/generic/pragmatic qualitative research, which involves using an eclectic approach taken up to best match the research question at hand. This is often called the mixed-method approach.
2. Ethnographic Research. An example of applied ethnographic research is the study of a particular culture and their understanding of the role of a particular disease in their cultural framework.
3. Grounded Theory is an inductive type of research, based or "grounded" in the observations or data from which it was developed; it uses a variety of data sources, including quantitative data, review of records, interviews, observation and surveys.
4. Phenomenology describes the "subjective reality" of an event, as perceived by the study population; it is the study of a phenomenon.
5. Biographical Research is aligned to the social interpretive paradigm of research and is concerned with the reconstruction of life histories and the constitution of meaning based on biographical narratives and documents. The starting point for this approach is the understanding of an individual biography in terms of its social constitution, as influenced by symbolic interactionism, phenomenological sociology of knowledge (Alfred Schütz, Peter L. Berger, and Thomas Luckmann), and ethnomethodology (Harold Garfinkel).

6. Philosophical Research is conducted by field experts within the boundaries of a specific field of study or profession, the best qualified individual in any field of study to use an intellectual analysis, in order to clarify definitions, identify ethics, or make a value judgment concerning an issue in their field of study their lives.
7. Critical Social Research, used by a researcher to understand how people communicate and develop symbolic meanings.
8. Ethical Inquiry, an intellectual analysis of ethical problems. It includes the study of ethics as related to obligation, rights, duty, right and wrong, choice etc.
9. Social Science and Governmental Research to understand social services, government operations, and recommendations (or not) regarding future developments and programs, including whether or not government should be involved.
10. Activist Research which aims to raise the views of the underprivileged or "underdogs" to prominence to the elite or master classes, the latter who often control the public view or positions.
11. Foundational Research, examines the foundations for a science, analyzes the beliefs, and develops ways to specify how a knowledge base should change in light of new information.
12. Historical Research allows one to discuss past and present events in the context of the present condition, and allows one to reflect and provide possible answers to current issues and problems. Historical research helps us in answering questions such as: Where have we come from, where are we, who are we now and where are we going?
13. Visual Ethnography. It uses visual methods of data collection, including photo, voice, photo elicitation, collaging, drawing, and mapping. These techniques have been used extensively as a participatory qualitative technique and to make the familiar strange.
14. Autoethnography, the study of self, is a method of qualitative research in which the researcher uses their personal experience to address an issue.

Data Analysis

Interpretive techniques

As a form of qualitative inquiry, students of interpretive inquiry (interpretivists) often disagree with the idea of theory-free observation or knowledge. Whilst this crucial philosophical realization is also held by researchers in other fields, interpretivists are often the most aggressive in taking this philosophical realization to its logical conclusions. For example, an interpretivist researcher might believe in the existence of an objective reality 'out there', but argue that the social and educational reality we act on the basis of never allows a single human subject to directly access the reality 'out there' in reality (this is a view shared by constructivist philosophies).

To researchers outside the qualitative research field, the most common analysis of qualitative data is often perceived to be observer impression. That is, expert or bystander observers examine the data, interpret it via forming an impression and report their impression in a structured and sometimes quantitative form.

Coding

In general, coding refers to the act of associating meaningful ideas with the data of interest. In the context of qualitative research, interpretative aspects of the coding process are often explicitly recognized, articulated, and celebrated; producing specific words or short phrases believed to be useful abstractions over the data.

As an act of sense making, most coding requires the qualitative analyst to read the data and demarcate segments within it, which may be done at multiple and different times throughout the data analysis process. Each segment is labeled with a 'code' – usually a word or short phrase suggesting how the associated data segments inform the research objectives. In contrast with more quantitative forms of coding, mathematical ideas and forms are usually under-developed in a 'pure' qualitative data analysis. When coding is complete, the analyst may prepare reports via a mix of: summarizing the prevalence of codes, discussing similarities and differences in related codes across distinct original sources/contexts, or comparing the relationship between one or more codes.

Some qualitative data that is highly structured (e.g., open-ended responses from surveys or tightly defined interview questions) is typically coded with minimal additional segmentation of the data. Quantitative analysis based on codes from statistical theory is typically the capstone analytical step for this type of qualitative data. A common form of coding is open-ended coding, while other more structured techniques such as axial coding or integration have also been described and articulated (Strauss & Corbin, 1990).Because qualitative analyses are often more inductive than the hypothesis testing nature of most quantitative research, the existing 'theoretical sensitivity' (i.e., familiarity with established theories in the field) of the analyst becomes a more pressing concern in producing an acceptable analysis.

Contemporary qualitative data analyses are often supported by computer programs (termed Computer Assisted Qualitative Data Analysis Software) used with or without the detailed hand coding and labeling of the past decades. These programs do not supplant the interpretive nature of coding, but rather are aimed at enhancing analysts' efficiency at applying, retrieving, and storing the codes generated from reading the data. Many programs enhance efficiency in editing and revision of codes, which allow for more effective work sharing, peer review, recursive examination of data, and analysis of large datasets.

Common Qualitative Data Analysis Software includes:

- MAXQDA (mixed methods)
- QDA MINER
- ATLAS.ti
- Dedoose (mixed methods)
- NVivo

A frequent criticism of quantitative coding approaches is against the transformation of qualitative data into predefined (nomothetic) data structures, underpinned by 'objective properties'; the variety, richness, and individual characteristics of the qualitative data is argued to be largely omitted from such data coding processes, rendering the original collection of qualitative data somewhat pointless.

To defend against the criticism of too much subjective variability in the categories and relationships identified from data, qualitative analysts respond by thoroughly articulating their definitions of codes and linking those codes soundly to the underlying data, thereby preserving some of the richness that might be absent from a mere list of codes, whilst satisfying the need for repeatable procedure held by experimentally oriented researchers.

RECURSIVE ABSTRACTION

As defined by Leshan 2012, this is a method of qualitative data analysis where qualitative datasets are analyzed without coding. A common method here is recursive abstraction, where datasets are summarized; those summaries are therefore furthered into summary and so on. The end result is a more compact summary that would have been difficult to accurately discern without the preceding steps of distillation.

A frequent criticism of recursive abstraction is that the final conclusions are several times removed from the underlying data. While it is true that poor initial summaries will certainly yield an inaccurate final report, qualitative analysts can respond to this criticism. They do so, like those using coding method, by documenting the reasoning behind each summary step, citing examples from the data where statements were included and where statements were excluded from the intermediate summary.

Coding and "Thinking"

Some data analysis techniques rely on using computers to scan and reduce large sets of qualitative data. At their most basic level, numerical coding relies on counting words, phrases, or coincidences of tokens within the data; other similar techniques are the analyses of phrases and exchanges in conversational analyses. Often referred to as content analysis, a basic structural building block to conceptual analysis, the technique utilizes mixed methodology to unpack both small and large corpuses. Content analysis is frequently used in sociology to explore relationships, such as the change in perceptions of race over time (Morning 2008), or the lifestyles of temporal contractors (Evans, et al. 2004).Content analysis techniques thus help to provide broader output for a larger, more accurate conceptual analysis.

Mechanical techniques are particularly well-suited for a few scenarios. One such scenario is for datasets that are simply too large for a human to effectively analyze, or where analysis of them would be cost prohibitive relative to the value of information they contain. Another scenario is when the chief value of a dataset is the extent to which it contains "red flags" (e.g., searching for reports of certain adverse events within a lengthy journal dataset from patients in a clinical trial) or "green flags" (e.g., searching for mentions of your brand in positive reviews of marketplace products). Many researchers would consider these procedures on their data sets to be misuse of their data collection and purposes.

A frequent criticism of mechanical techniques is the absence of a human interpreter; computer analysis is relatively new having arrived in the late 1980s to the university sectors. And while masters of these methods are able to write sophisticated software to mimic some human decisions, the bulk of the "analysis" is still nonhuman. Analysts respond by proving the value of their methods relative to either a) hiring and training a human team to analyze the data or b) by letting the data go untouched, leaving any actionable nuggets undiscovered; almost all coding schemes indicate probably studies for further research.

Data sets and their analyses must also be written up, reviewed by other researchers, circulated for comments, and finalized for public review. Numerical coding must be available in the published articles, if the methodology and findings are to be compared across research studies in traditional literature review and recommendation formats.

Distinct Qualitative Paradigms

Contemporary qualitative research has been conducted using a large number of paradigms that influence conceptual and metatheoretical concerns of legitimacy, control, data analysis, ontology, and epistemology, among others. Qualitative research conducted in the twenty-first century has been characterized by a distinct turn toward more interpretive, postmodern, and critical practices. Guba and Lincoln (2005) identify five main paradigms of contemporary qualitative research: positivism, postpositivism, critical theories, constructivism, and participatory/cooperative paradigms. Each of the paradigms listed by Guba and Lincoln are characterized by axiomatic differences in axiology, intended action/impact of research, control of research process/outcomes, relationship to foundations of truth and knowledge, validity and trust (see below), textual representation and voice of the researcher and research participants, and commensurability with other paradigms. In particular, commensurability involves the extent to which concerns from 2 paradigms e.g., "can be retrofitted to each other in ways that make the simultaneous practice of both possible". Positivist and post positivist paradigms share commensurable assumptions, but are largely incommensurable with critical, constructivist, and participatory paradigms of research and knowledge. Likewise, critical, constructivist, and participatory paradigms are commensurable on certain issues (e.g., the intended action and textual representation of research).

Qualitative research in the 2000s has also been characterized by concern with everyday categorization and ordinary storytelling. This "narrative turn" is producing an enormous literature as researchers present sensitizing concepts and perspectives that bear especially on narrative practice, which centers on the circumstances and communicative actions of storytelling. Catherine Riessman (1993) and Gubrium and Holstein (2009) provide analytic strategies, and Holstein and Gubrium (2012) present the variety of approaches in recent comprehensive texts. More recent developments in narrative practice has increasingly taken up the issue of institutional conditioning of such practices (see Gubrium and Holstein 2000).

However, not all scholars agree on the usefulness of paradigms. A critical view of understanding qualitative inquiry vis-à-vis paradigms has been recently put forth by Pernecky (2016), who has argued that problems arise when paradigms are "interpreted in a rigid fashion and compartmentalized into static schemata" (p. 18). It is therefore more fruitful to think in terms of flows and continuums, and even embrace a post-paradigmatic qualitative research. In his words:

"The problem with laying down prescriptive rules about what qualitative research is and how it ought to proceed lies in the narrowing of the possibilities of an abundant and constantly devolving body of philosophical thought. When we accept paradigms uncritically as the 'givens', qualitative knowledge becomes habituated, and paradigms grow into hegemonic systems of organization (Pernecky, 2016, p. 194)".

Trustworthiness

A central issue in qualitative research is trustworthiness (also known as credibility, or in quantitative studies, validity). There are many different ways of establishing trustworthiness, including: member check, interviewer corroboration, peer debriefing, prolonged engagement, negative case analysis, auditability, confirmability, bracketing, and balance. Most of these methods are described in Lincoln and Guba (1985). As exemplified by researchers Preston Teeter and Jorgen Sandberg, data triangulation and eliciting examples of interviewee accounts are two of the most commonly used methods of establishing trustworthiness in qualitative studies. Dependability is equivalent to the notion of reliability in quantitative methods and is the extent to which two or more people are likely to come to the same conclusions by examining the same evidence. Again, Lincoln and Guba (1985) is the salient reference.

DATA COLLECTION

In qualitative research, the researcher is the primary data collection instrument. Qualitative research involves data collected from participant observations, interviews, questionnaires, phone calls, focus groups etc. Interviewing, focus groups, and participant observation are common modes of qualitative data gathering. Interviews are used in most types of qualitative research. Participant observation is a method particularly employed by ethnographers in the anthropological tradition. It is used to learn about the naturally occurring routines, interactions and practices of a particular group of people in their social environments, and so to understand their culture. When a researcher becomes a part of the participants in the situation under observation, it is called a participant observer. Furthermore, qualitative data can be used to strengthen quantitative research designs in general and intervention research designs (i.e., experimental, quasi-experimental) in particular. For example, in educational psychology, researchers could conduct a qualitative pilot study to determine which group of students should be selected for quantitative study by observing or interviewing different groups of students.

Focus Groups

Focus group discussion in qualitative method has gained popularity across the social sciences over the past decade. Prior to the late 1970s, focus groups were mainly used in marketing and studies in the field of business. They have become more popular in many fields including education, communication, media studies, feminist research, sociology and social psychology. Focus groups are also known as 'group interviews'. The members are encouraged to interact and have discussions. The data collected by focus group discussion are seldom produced through interview and observation; it enlightens us with its power of knowledge. Focus group discussion also focuses on the process beyond the individual's memory and desires. The richness and complexity of group dynamics should be considered. Focus group can also access to social interactional dynamics that produce particular memories, ideologies, and practices among the group members. It themselves becomes relevant, termed as units of analysis of our study. Questions, issues and topics process focus group. Through different dynamics multiple angles of vision can be seen in the new world in unexpected ways. Focus groups help us move towards constructing a 'methodology of getting lost" and toward enacting "double practices" (lather, 2001). This seems a necessary step towards conducting qualitative research. Keeping norms and rules of groups in mind the researcher and research participants realize that interpretation of individual are situated, provisional, contingent, unstable thus it's unchangeable. It is necessary for the researcher to have self-reflectivity that involves making the research transparent rhetorical and poetic work of the researcher in representing the object of the study. It is theoretically important to construct a mutual ground between the researcher and the research participants. The second sense of self-reflexivity is important to encourage refection on interpretive research as the dual practice of knowledge gathering and self transformation is done through self-reflection and mutual reflection. Allowing ourselves to dwell in the existing inevitable indeterminacies, we are leading ourselves in the best way of the qualitative research practice.

According to Lederman, a focus group is a 'technique that involves the use of profound group interviews in which participants are selected because they are a purposive sampling of a specific population, with the group being 'focused' on a given topic'. (Rabiee, 2004). According to Powell et al., a group of individuals selected and gathered by researchers to discuss and comment on, from personal experience, the topic that is the subject of the research form a focus group.(Gibbs, 1997)

Some of the features of focus group discussions include, member's involvement, a number of consecutive meetings, the common characteristics of members with respect to interests, the evolvement of qualitative data, and discussion within the group that is focused on a topic, that is determined by the purposes of the research(Freitas, 1998). In other words, a focus group is an informal discussion among a group of selected individuals about a particular topic (Wilkinson 2004). A focus group, as a research method, involves more than one participant per data collection session.

Some of the main characteristics of Focus Groups are; Focus groups involve people in which there is a group of usually 4-10 members. The group size depends on the topic. It should be understood that the size should be small enough so that all the members get a chance to share their views and yet, large enough for people to get different perspectives (Ogunbameru, 2003).Participants are homogenous and unfamiliar with each other which means that people who have similar ages, ethnic backgrounds, etc. this is because it will help the session very effectively as there won't be too many clashes. It should be noted that the group should not be too homogenous because some amount of heterogeneity is required to get useful information when it comes to recalling past events or religious groups (Ogunbameru, 2003).Focus groups are a data collection procedure where in, the main purpose is to determine the perception, feelings, and manner of thinking. These are not aimed to develop consensus or to arrive at some agreeable plan (Ogunbameru, 2003). Focus groups make use of Qualitative data, which means that the data is collected using qualitative tools, which requires very skilled people. This data provides a great insight into the phenomenological world of the members, taking into consideration the attitude, perceptions, and thoughts (Ogunbameru, 2003). Focus groups have a focused discussion where in the leader maintains focus on a particular topic. This helps the discussion to stay on track as every member has different ideas to pool in about the same topic (Ogunbameru, 2003).

The significance of focus group methodology is that it helps in exploring what people perceive and think, and understanding why the members have certain opinions about what they believe in(n.d, 2009). Jenny Kitzinger (2005), a famous focus group researcher, is of the opinion that focus group method is an 'ideal' approach for examining the stories, experiences, points of view, beliefs, needs and concerns of individuals. Working in a group enables the researchers to receive different communication forms that the members use in their day-today interactions with other. These communications and interactions involve joking, arguing, teasing and recapturing past events. This is important since it may not be easy, or even possible to receive the knowledge and attitudes of various people while they respond to more direct form of questions

One of the main purposes of focus group discussion is to get light into the respondents' phenomenological world of experience, thinking, perceiving and feeling.

These experiences, feelings, attitudes might be independent of a group or its cultural and social settings but are more likely to reveal itself in the interaction with other people in a group or another social setting. Focus group discussions help in elaborating the different viewpoints and emotional processes of each member within a group context. The individual interview is simpler for the researcher to control in comparison to a focus group discussion. A focus group discussion, in comparison to other methods helps the research to gain larger pool information in a much lesser amount of time. This observation depends on waiting for things to happen, whereas the researcher has to follow an interview guide in a focus group. In this aspect, focus group discussions are not natural but organized and planned. These discussions are especially helpful when there are differences related to power between its members, decision-makers or professionals, when the culture and language of a specific group is of, and when the researcher or a member wants to understand and explore the level of consensus over a given theme or topic(Kreuger, 1993).

Role of the Leader

Pre-session Strategy refers to the leader's ability to understand the importance of small talk just prior to group discussion. The facilitator must cordially greet the group members and begin small talk while at the same time avoid the topics and issues that will be discussed during the sessions. This will allow the group leader to observe the kind of interactions and understand which participant has what qualities. Recording is beneficial for the leader via tape recording and note taking. Note taking is useful as they can be utilized even if the tape recorder stops working. Someone other than the group leader or the facilitator should take detailed and in depth notes of the discussion. Beginning of the Discussion includes the usual pattern of discussion which is welcome, overview and topic, ground rules and first question. The overview must provide an explanation of the purpose and importance of the topic of discussion. Ground rules must be stated explicitly. Some of the examples are, minimizing or eliminating side conversations, one person talks at a time, no criticizing what others have to say and treating everyone's opinion with respect and dignity. The initial conversation should include an "ice breaker" in order to make the members more comfortable and open.

Pause and probe is the skill of the moderator to give each participant a chance to jump in. As a general rule, a moderator should pause for at least five seconds after a participant talks or before beginning to talk. Probes, such as "would you explain that further?" or "Would you give me an example?" help to give additional information. Being prepared for the unexpected is one of the abilities of the focus group leaders in order for the efficient functioning of the groups. Some examples of unexpected events are no one showing up (make sure you bring list and phone numbers), only a few showing up (hold group anyway), meeting place is inadequate for the members to reach, the group members get too involved and don't want to leave (have formal ending), bad or hazardous weather (call everyone and cancel).

Organization Skills helps focus group leaders to plan the theme for group discussions and also develop a printed outline for the meetings. There may be more productive discussions when every member of the focus group has a copy of the printed agenda before starting the discussion. This allows the member to have some time to review the topics and focus on key relevant issues. The leader should use the counseling skills in order for the discussion to take place effectively.

Listening and Note Taking enables the focus group leaders must have highly developed listening skills in order to guide the group discussions by keeping focus on what each person is saying, while at the same time take notes during the discussion. The leader must narrow down to a single focus instead of looking at all the aspects spoken during the discussion. The leader focuses on similar phrases and words to narrow down the discussion to a single topic.

Rephrasing refers to skills in which leader repeats what others are saying for more clarification during a group discussion. The focus group leader typically asks group members for more in-depth opinions after rephrasing. It allows group members to have a broad perspective in order to view topics from different angles and interpretations. Emotional Control refers to the group leader's ability to control his or her emotions in order for the discussion to be effective. It requires developing a tough skin to be able to take on the lead in the discussion when people lose their tempers. Leaders must aim to diffuse anger and redirect the emotions with constructive analysis and suggestions. S/he must allow providing an avenue to release all the emotions within constructively. After dealing with emotions, the leader must redirect the focus of group discussion.

Moderating Skills makes a group leader understand and regulate the unofficial roles assumed by all the group members during the discussion and use the members to help solve group problems. For example, the role of the "tension reducer" is to help the members to resolve conflicts and differences in order to reduce anxiety, while the "task master" helps the members to focus on the purpose of the meeting. Group moderators must be mentally alert, listen well, and think quickly in order to have an effective group discussion. All the questions must be memorized and handy for the leader. Concluding the focus group is necessary for the focus group leader in order to get a formal ending of the session. The leader must thank the group members for participating in the session and summarize what was discussed during the session. S/he should ask if something was missed out in the summary of the session. This helps the group members to have an exact idea of what happened in the session and have something to take along.

How to Conduct Focus Group Discussions

For the purpose of conducting an FGD where the topic being discussed is of sensitive nature, it is recommended that the participants be of same sex, age range and socio economic background. The trainers should preferably also be of the same sex, if the topic of discussion is sensitive. It is also desirable that the participants do not know each other prior to the discussion. The samples are chosen purposively. (Odimegwu, 2000)

Informed consent must be taken before beginning the discussion where the members should be briefed about the topic of discussion, informed about their rights, confidentiality and that their identities will not be revealed in any report or publication. (Toolkit for Conducting Focus Groups)

An important consideration to keep in mind is the homogeneity of the group members and settings and the nature of open-ended questions which will drive the members to talk more freely from the constraints they might feel during a personal interview. (Odimegwu, 2000) The discussion must be held in a relaxed and natural setting or environment, with the entire session recorded (audio or visual). There should also be a note-taker who jots down all the important aspects of the discussion but is not a part of the discussion. This note-taker must have in-depth knowledge about the issue at hand and should be trained in observing verbal and non verbal feedback, example facial expressions. It is his duty to translate the notes taken during session into data that is the used for analysis. (Odimegwu, 2000) Areas of interest to be discussed during the session need to be chalked out by the moderators and organizers prior to the session and then, it is the duty of the moderator to make sure that all these areas are covered during the discussion. The moderator directs the conversation and encourages participation to ensure richness of discussion and data. It is the duty of the moderator to introduce new topics and have an unbiased approach throughout the discussion. (Odimegwu, 2000)

Literature provides a basic groundwork and suggestions for conducting focus groups. According to Puchta and Potter (2004), it is very important to produce an informal environment in the group. The moderator should facilitate in creating a liberal environment encouraging members to share and put forth their views and keeping track of the flow of the session, preventing them from drifting from the topic of discussion. (Flick, 2006) Often the participants do not know each other, and so, it is the job of the moderator to ensure that everyone feels comfortable and there is a good rapport. The purpose and format of the discussion of the discussion should be conveyed in the beginning of the session. All participants should be encouraged to participate, share their views and be told that divergent views are also welcome. (Toolkit for Conducting Focus Groups)

Flick (2006) says that a formal explanation of the procedure is given to the participants. Expectation setting is an essential component in this step. Expectations can be being involved in the discussion, argue about certain topics, collective problem solving. Introducing the members to one another and warming up are necessary to prepare them for the discussion. Here, the moderator establishes and conveys the common grounds of the members to facilitate or reinforce community feeling. The actual discussion takes place following "discussion stimuli", which may be in the form of a provocative thesis, a short film, lecture on a text, or unfolding of a concrete problem for which a solution needs to be found. In groups where the members do not know one another in advance, phases of strangeness with, of orientation to, adaptation to, and familiarity with the group as well as conformity and the discussion drying up are gone through. The questions must be open ended and there should be a smooth transition in the type of questions asked through the course of the discussion. The session should ideally start with introductory questions to address the general topic, helping the participants to understand the broader context of the issue, followed by key questions designed to address the specific information, and ending with questions aimed to summarize the opinion of all the participants. (Magloff)

Advantages and Disadvantages of Focus Group Discussions

Focus groups data collection method has several advantages in conducting a qualitative research. The following are various advantages of using a focus group to obtain data.

There is flexibility of the focus group research in being used as a qualitative method or a combination of the former with quantitative techniques (n.d., HCC Education Digital Library).The moderator is permitted to inquire into and examine unforeseen issues due to this kind of format. Has high face validity and naturalistic- as it includes storytelling, joking, disagreements, boasting and more (n.d., HCC Education Digital Library & Morgan). It is relatively inexpensive/relatively low cost (n.d., HCC Education Digital Library). Provides relatively fast results (n.d., HCC Education Digital Library).Consumes lesser time unlike structured interviews in order to increase sample sizes and resource investment (n.d., HCC Education Digital Library). It is helpful and important for needs assessment and project evaluation projects (Savithiri, 2009).Regarding the facts and numbers in research, meaning behind these facts can also be found and confirmed through surveys as it is qualitative in nature(Savithiri, 2009). It is relatively simple to carry out (n.d., National Center for Postsecondary Improvement). It consumes less time as large sample size can be studied (n.d., National Center for Postsecondary Improvement).Information is gained from group interaction due to group dynamics (n.d., National Center for Postsecondary Improvement). It helps in obtaining and gathering contracted and incisive data of specific topic (Morgan).Many new perspectives and opinions are obtained which results in insights (Morgan). Sensitive topics can be discussed leading to personal disclosures (Silverman, 2004).Often these interactions result in creating 'synergistic effects' (Silverman, 2004).Vocabulary and language used can be observed (Silverman, 2004). It is much more efficient when the data being gathered is very much related to the researcher's interests(Morgan).The moderator keeps the discussion in sync with the topic and makes sure one individual does not dominate the other; hence follows an 'egalitarian' method(Silverman, 2004 & n.d., Focus Groups: Issues Regarding Advantages and Disadvantages). Non-verbal behavior as well plays a role in the moderator's decision making and research results (n.d., Focus Groups: Issues Regarding Advantages and Disadvantages). High possibilities in resulting in rich and in-depth information or data (n.d., Focus Groups: Issues Regarding Advantages and Disadvantages & Deem, 1997). It is useful for exploratory research (Deem, 1997). Group interaction can be observed in a controlled setting(Deem, 1997). The reactions of participants towards each other can be analyzed (n.d., Southalabama Education: Strengths and Weaknesses of Focus Groups). Previously neglected or unnoticed phenomena can be drawn towards the researcher's attention(Silverman, 2004).Helps to inform the development of survey instruments(Silverman, 2004).Opportunistic use of focus groups results in improvised research design and impoverished data(Silverman, 2004).

Though focus groups method of data collection has several advantages; the limitations of the same cannot be ignored. Has less experimental control(n.d., HCC Education Digital Library).Data collected is usually difficult to analyze; as the discussion must be audio or video taped, field notes to be recorded and the verbatim to be transcribed (n.d., HCC Education Digital Library & Savithiri, 2009).Requires or the need for carefully trained interviewers(n.d., HCC Education Digital Library).Groups may vary considerably. Groups may be difficult to assemble (n.d., HCC Education Digital Library).Discussion must be conducted in an environment that is conducive to conversation (n.d., HCC Education Digital Library). There is high potential for leading and bias (n.d., Focus Groups: Issues Regarding Advantages and Disadvantages). Moderator or rather the facilitation of the discussion may be critical as the group largely banks on the assisted discussion in order to produce results(Savithiri, 2009).The need for skilled and trained moderators or interviewers is necessary (n.d., HCC Education Digital Library).There is a high chance or risk for the moderator to dominate or 'hijack' the discussion(Savithiri, 2009). There may be difficulties in terms of the sample study results representing the population as participants are self-selected; hence generalization becomes difficult or impossible(Savithiri, 2009).The moderator may influence the group interactions thus distorting results or findings (Morgan). Participant's involvement and contribution in the discussion also plays a major role(Morgan).Issues may arise if topics are controversial in nature leading to disagreements and arguments (Morgan). Results obtained may be biased as one or two prevalent people may influence the interaction or discussion(n.d., Focus Groups: Issues Regarding Advantages and Disadvantages).Dealing with sensitive topics is a challenge(n.d., Focus Groups: Issues Regarding Advantages and Disadvantages).Contrived or artificial environment also may influence the interactions and responses, thus leading to biased results (n.d., Focus Groups: Issues Regarding Advantages and Disadvantages).Ethical issues may rise regarding confidentiality aspect (Deem, 1997). Measurement validity may be low(n.d., Southalabama Education: Strengths and Weaknesses of Focus Groups)

DATAANALYSIS

Qualitative data analysis contains reviewing, summarizing, generalizing and interpreting data in an appropriate and accurate way. It is to describe and explain the phenomena or social worlds being studied. One of the most important steps in the qualitative research process is analysis of data. Analyzing qualitative data also requires researchers' patience. There are two different analytical procedures: Meaning and discovery-Focused approaches. Meaning-focused approaches emphasize meaning comprehension. In other words, try to understand the subjective meaning of experiences for the participants, instead of placing those meanings into researchers' own conceptions. Discovery-focused techniques aim to establish patterns and connections among elements of data. However, no matter which procedure is used, it is essential to apply an effective system for retrieving data because of the identity of qualitative data analysis, which is exploring data progressively.

There are also a variety of the available analysis tools and strategies for qualitative data analysis.

1. Constant Comparison Analysis, or called "coding system" : Coding enables the researcher to locate and bring together similarly labeled data for examination and to retrieve data related to more than one label when wanting to consider patterns, connections, or distinctions between them.
2. Keywords-in-Context: It is a data analysis method that reveals how respondents use words in context by comparing words that appear before and after "key words. KWIC is a helpful analysis to utilize when there are specific words that are of interest to the researcher or when the data appear to be less rich in information.
3. Word Count: Word counts are based on the belief that all people have distinctive vocabulary and word usage patterns.
4. Classical Content Analysis: Classical content analysis is similar to constant comparison analysis and also is used frequently in qualitative research.
5. Domain Analysis: Domain analysis represents a search for the larger units of cultural knowledge, which Spradley (1979) called domains. This method of analysis stems from the belief that symbols are an important way of communicating cultural meaning. This analysis should be used when researchers are interested in understanding relationships among concepts.
6. Taxonomic Analysis: Taxonomic analysis is the second step after domain analysis. This analysis helps the researcher to understand how participants are using specific words.
7. Componential Analysis: Componential analysis is another step that can be undertaken after domains are created. It is used when a researcher is trying to uncover relationships between words.

Using Computers in Qualitative Data Analysis

There are many computer programs are available to help in analyzing qualitative data. The capacity of computers to effectively sort, store and retrieve information makes their use in qualitative data analysis appealing. However, it is important to notice that computers can only aid in some parts of analysis; computer software do not code data or replace the conceptual processes. It cannot analyse qualitative data for the researcher.

Qualitative research methodologies are oriented towards developing understanding of the meaning and experience dimensions of human lives and their social worlds. Good qualitative research is characterized by congruence between the perspective that informs the research questions and the research methods used.

5

The Basics of Pharmaceutical Market Research

The pharmaceutical industry is a multi-billion dollar business tasked with researching, developing, manufacturing and distributing drugs for human and animal use. The stakes are high; lives and money are on the line each time a new medicine is conceived. And because the process from drug conception to its delivery is a long one, it's important that companies do the necessary research to insure that they are meeting a worthy demand and have the requisite tools and information that they need to succeed. Otherwise, they risk losing a lot of money and a lot of time on a product that no one wants or needs. Combine that with the changing landscape of the pharma industry – this point in time of American drug history when key drug patents are expiring (typically after a 20 year period) and more and more generics are hitting the market – and it's easy to understand that pharmaceutical companies must find new drugs, as well as boost declining sales of their established ones, if they want to survive.

Identify Consumer Need

Big pharma doesn't just serve patients, it also serves a host of other types of consumers, from the clinicians who prescribe drugs and the hospitals that buy and administer them to the distributors and pharmacies that stock and deliver them. With so many customer types, it's paramount that drug companies learn as much as possible about each one so that they can identify the areas and people with the most profitable issues to address. They can do this through a variety of research measures. They can use established secondary research literature or conduct primary research (such as ethnographic studies and satisfaction surveys with physicians, hospitals and/or patients) themselves.

Assess the Market

Picking the right environment (both physically and generally) in which to market a drug is critical. Disease patterns, political turmoil, economic stability, as well as market size/segmentation and operating conditions, are just a few of the key factors affecting a company's overall success with a product. Pharmaceutical market research can highlight any obstacles or opportunities that might disturb or encourage favorable outcomes.

Provide a Competitive Analysis

Emerging new products to the market are only one type of threat. Generic products can also severely impact a company's bottom line. Thus, it's imperative that pharmaceutical companies keep on top of the products that their competitors are developing, as well as improving. They can utilize SWOT analyses and sales force assessments to diagnose and treat deficiencies. Focus groups and interviews can be used to expose untapped technological innovations and other resources. Competitive analysis can save companies from reinventing the wheel. They can observe and use others' successes for their own benefit instead.

Address Compliance and Other Regulatory Concerns

The pharmaceutical industry is strictly regulated. It must deal with patient and data privacy issues and comply with FDA and patent regulations. Pharmaceutical market research can help companies monitor developing patent laws and any changes to FDA legislation and gather consumer feedback so that they can protect or modify their practices as needed.

Update Shareholders

A good pharmaceutical market research project can reveal industry trends and help forecast market growth. It can describe how well a company is (or is not) doing with its consumer encounters, marketing efforts and distribution methods. It can provide the raw data needed for accurate benchmarking, and it can uncover unmet needs. These facts assist shareholders, who use them to focus and direct decisions, shaping their business's future.

Market research started to be conceptualized and put into formal practice during the 1930s, as an offshoot of the advertising boom of the Golden Age of radio in the United States. Advertisers began to realize the significance of demographics revealed by sponsorship of different radio programs.

Market research For Business/Planning

Market research is a way of getting an overview of consumers' wants, needs and beliefs. It can also involve discovering how they act. The research can be used to determine how a product could be marketed. Peter Drucker believed market research to be the quintessence of marketing. Market research is a way that producers and the marketplace study the consumer and gather information about the consumers' needs. There are two major types of market research: primary research, which is sub-divided into quantitative and qualitativeresearch, and secondary research.

Factors that can be investigated through market research include:

- Market information: Through market information one can know the prices of different commodities in the market, as well as the supply and demand situation. Market researchers have a wider role than previously recognized by helping their clients to understand social, technical, and even legal aspects of markets.
- Market segmentation: Market segmentation is the division of the market or population into subgroups with similar motivations. It is widely used for segmenting on geographic differences, demographic differences (age, gender, ethnicity, etc.), technographic differences, psychographic differences, and differences in product use. For B2B segmentation firmographics is commonly used.
- Market trends: Market trends are the upward or downward movement of a market, during a period of time. Determining the market size may be more difficult if one is starting with a new innovation. In this case, you will have to derive the figures from the number of potential customers, or customer segments.
- SWOT analysis: SWOT is a written analysis of the Strengths, Weaknesses, Opportunities and Threats to a business entity. A SWOT may also be written up for the competition to understand how to develop the marketing and product mixes.

Another factor that can be measured is marketing effectiveness. This includes:

- Customer analysis (Segmentation of target customers)
- Choice modelling
- Competitor analysis
- Risk analysis
- Product research
- Advertisement research
- Marketing mix modeling
- Simulated test marketing

Influence from the Internet

The availability of research by way of the Internet has influenced a vast number of consumers using this media; for gaining knowledge relating to virtually every type of available product and service. It has been added to by the growth factor of emerging global markets, such as China, Indonesia and Russia, which is significantly exceeding that of the established and more advanced B2B e-commerce markets. Various statistics show that the increasing demands of consumers are reflected not only in the wide and varied range of general Internet researching applications, but in online shopping research penetration.

This is stimulated by product-enhancing websites, graphics, and content designed to attract casual "surfing" shoppers, researching for their particular needs, competitive prices and quality. According to the Small Business Administration (SBA), a successful business is significantly contributed to by gaining knowledge about customers, competitors, and the associated industry. Market research creates not only this understanding, but is the process of data analysis regarding which products and services are in demand.

The convenience and easy accessibility of the Internet has created a global B2C e-commerce research facility, for a vast online shopping network that has motivated retail markets in developed countries. In 2010 between US$400 billion and $600 billion in revenue was generated by this medium. It was anticipated that in 2015 this online market w generate between $700 billion and $950 billion.

Beyond online web-based market research activities, the Internet has also influenced high-street modes of data collection by, for example, replacing the traditional paper clipboardwith online survey providers. Over the last 5 years, mobile surveys have become increasingly popular. Mobile has opened the door to innovative new methods of engaging respondents, such as social voting communities.

Research and Social Media Applications

The UK Market Research Society (MRS) reports research has shown that on average, the three social media platforms primarily used by Millennials are LinkedIn, Facebook and YouTube. Social Media applications, according to T-Systems, help generate the B2B E-commerce market and develop electronic business process efficiency. This application is a highly effective vehicle for market research, which combined with E-commerce, is now regarded as a separate, extremely profitable field of global business. While many B2B business models are being updated, the various advantages and benefits offered by Social Media platforms are being integrated within them.

Business intelligence organization have compiled a comprehensive report related to global online retail sales, defining continued growth patterns and trends in the industry. Headed "Global B2C E-Commerce and Online Payment Market 2014" the report perceives a decrease in overall growth rates in North America and Western Europe, as the expected growth in the online market sales, is absorbed into the emerging markets. It is forecast that the Asia-Pacific region will see the fastest growth in the B2C E-Commerce market and replace North America as the B2C E-Commerce sales region leader, within a few years. This effectively, offers a significant, motivational platform for new Internet services, to promote user market research-friendly applications.

Research and Market Sectors

The primary online sale providers in B2C E-Commerce, worldwide, includes the USA based Amazon.com Inc. which remains the E-Commerce revenues, global leader. The growth leaders in the world top ten are two online companies from China, both of which conducted Initial Public Offering (IPO) this year; Alibaba Group Holding Ltd. and JD Inc. Another company from the top ten is Cnova N.V., a recently formed E-Commerce subsidiary of the French Group Casino, with various store retailers developing and expanding their E-Commerce facilities worldwide. It is a further indication of how consumers are increasingly being attracted to the opportunities of online researching and expanding their awareness of what is available to them.

Service providers; for example those related to finance, foreign market trade and investment promote a variety of information and research opportunities to online users. In addition, they provide comprehensive and competitive strategies with market research tools, designed to promote worldwide business opportunities for entrepreneurs and established providers. General access, to accurate and supported market research facilities, is a critical aspect of business development and success today. The Marketing Research Association was founded in 1957 and is recognized as one of the leading and prominent associations in the opinion and marketing research profession. It serves the purpose of providing insights and intelligence that helps businesses make decisions regarding the provision of products and services to consumers and industries.

This organization knowledge of market conditions and competition is gained by researching relevant sectors, which provide advantages for entry into new and established industries. It enables effective strategies to be implemented; the assessment of global environments in the service sectors, as well as foreign market trade and investment barriers! Research, is utilized for promoting export opportunities and inward investment, helping determine how to execute competitive strategies, focus on objective policies and strengthen global opportunities. It is a medium that influences, administrates and enforces agreements, preferences, leveling trading environments and competitiveness in the international marketplace.

The retail industry aspect of online market research, is being transformed worldwide by M-Commerce with its mobile audience, rapidly increasing as the volume and varieties of products purchased on the mobile medium, increases. Researches conducted in the markets of North America and Europe, revealed that the M-Commerce penetration on the total online retail trade, had attained 10%, or more. It was also shown that in emerging markets, smart-phone and tablet penetration is fast increasing and contributing significantly to online shopping growth.

Marketing research is "the process or set of processes that links the producers, customers, and end users to the marketer through information used to identify and define marketing opportunities and problems; generate, refine, and evaluate marketing actions; monitor marketing performance; and improve understanding of marketing as a process. Marketing research specifies the information required to address these issues, designs the method for collecting information, manages and implements the data collection process, analyzes the results, and communicates the findings and their implications."

It is the systematic gathering, recording, and analysis of qualitative and quantitative data about issues relating to marketing products and services. The goal of marketing research is to identify and assess how changing elements of the marketing mix impacts customer behavior. The term is commonly interchanged with market research; however, expert practitioners may wish to draw a distinction, in that market research is concerned specifically with markets, while marketing research is concerned specifically about marketing processes.Overview

Marketing research is often partitioned into two sets of categorical pairs, either by target market:

- Consumer marketing research, and
- Business-to-business (B2B) marketing research.

Or, alternatively, by methodological approach:

- Qualitative marketing research, and
- Quantitative marketing research.

Consumer marketing research is a form of applied sociology that concentrates on understanding the preferences, attitudes, and behaviors of consumers in a market-based economy, and it aims to understand the effects and comparative success of marketing campaigns. The field of consumer marketing research as a statistical science was pioneered by Arthur Nielsen with the founding of the ACNielsen Company in 1923.

Thus, marketing research may also be described as the systematic and objective identification, collection, analysis, and dissemination of information for the purpose of assisting management in decision making related to the identification and solution of problems and opportunities in marketing. The goal of market research is to obtain and provide management with viable information about the market (e.g. competitors), consumers, the product/service itself etc.

Role

The purpose of marketing research (MR) is to provide management with relevant, accurate, reliable, valid, and up to date market information. Competitive marketing environment and the ever-increasing costs attributed to poor decision making require that marketing research provide sound information. Sound decisions are not based on gut feeling, intuition, or even pure judgment.

Managers make numerous strategic and tactical decisions in the process of identifying and satisfying customer needs. They make decisions about potential opportunities, target market selection, market segmentation, planning and implementing marketing programs, marketing performance, and control. These decisions are complicated by interactions between the controllable marketing variables of product, pricing, promotion, and distribution. Further complications are added by uncontrollable environmental factors such as general economic conditions, technology, public policies and laws, political environment, competition, and social and cultural changes. Another factor in this mix is the complexity of consumers. Marketing research helps the marketing manager link the marketing variables with the environment and the consumers. It helps remove some of the uncertainty by providing relevant information about the marketing variables, environment, and consumers. In the absence of relevant information, consumers' response to marketing programs cannot be predicted reliably or accurately. Ongoing marketing research programs provide information on controllable and non-controllable factors and consumers; this information enhances the effectiveness of decisions made by marketing managers.

Traditionally, marketing researchers were responsible for providing the relevant information and marketing decisions were made by the managers. However, the roles are changing and marketing researchers are becoming more involved in decision making, whereas marketing managers are becoming more involved with research. The role of marketing research in managerial decision making is explained further using the framework of the DECIDE model.

History

Evidence for commercial research being gathered informally dates to the Medieval period. In 1380, the German textile manufacturer, Johann Fugger, travelled from Augsburg to Graben in order to gather information on the international textile industry. He exchanged detailed letters on trade conditions in relevant areas. Although, this type of information would have been termed "commercial intelligence" at the time, it created a precedent for the systemic collection of marketing information.

During the European age of discovery, industrial houses began to import exotic, luxury goods - calico cloth from India, porcelain, silk and tea from China, spices from India and South-East Asia and tobacco, sugar, rum and coffee from the New World. International traders began to demand information that could be used for marketing decisions. During this period, Daniel Defoe, a London merchant, published information on trade and economic resources of England and Scotland. Defoe was a prolific publisher and among his many publications are titles devoted to the state of trade including; Trade of Britain Stated, (1707); Trade of Scotland with France, (1713) and The Trade to India Critically and Calmly Considered, (1720) - all of which provided merchants and traders with important information on which to base business decisions.

Until the late 18th-century, European and North-American economies were characterised by local production and consumption. Produce, household goods and tools were produced by local artisans or farmers with exchange taking place in local markets or fairs. Under these conditions, the need for marketing information was minimail. However, the rise of mass-production following the industrial revolution, combined with improved transportation systems of the early 19th-century, led to the creation of national markets and ultimately, stimulated the need for more detailed information about customers, competitors, distribution systems and market communications.

By the 19th-century, manufacturers were exploring ways to understand the different market needs and behaviours of groups of consumers. A study of the German book trade found examples of both product differentiation and market segmentation as early as the 1820s. From the 1880s, German toy manufacturers were producing models of tin toys for specific geographic markets; London omnibuses and ambulances destined for the British market; French postal delivery vans for Continental Europe and American locomotives intended for sale in America. Such activities suggest that sufficient market information was collected to support detailed market segmentation.

In 1895, American advertising agency, N. H. Ayer & Son, used telegraph to contact publishers and state officials throughout the country about grain production, in an effort to construct an advertising schedule for client, Nichols-Shephard company, an agricultural machinery company in what many scholars believe is the first application of marketing research to solve a marketing/ advertising problem)

Between 1902 and 1910, George B Waldron, working at Mahin's Advertising Agency in the United States used tax registers, city directories and census data to show advertisers the proportion of educated vs illiterate consumers and the earning capacity of different occupations in a very early example of simple market segmentation. In 1911 Charles Coolidge Parlin was appointed as the Manager of the Commercial Research Division of the Advertising Department of the Curtis Publishing Company, thereby establishing the first in-house market research department - an event that has been described as marking the beginnings of organised marketing research. His aim was to turn market research into a science. Parlin published a number of studies of various product-markets including agriculture (1911); consumer goods (c.1911); department store lines (1912) a five-volume study of automobiles (1914).

In 1924 Paul Cherington improved on primitive forms of demographic market segmentation when he developed the 'ABCD' household typology; the first socio-demographic segmentation tool. By the 1930s, market researchers such as Ernest Dichter recognised that demographics alone were insufficient to explain different marketing behaviours and began exploring the use of lifestyles, attitudes, values, beliefs and culture to segment markets.

In the first three decades of the 20th-century, advertising agencies and marketing departments developed the basic techniques used in quantitative and qualitative research - survey methods, questionnaires, gallup polls etc. As early as

1901, Walter B Scott was undertaking experimental research for the Agate Club of Chicago. In 1910, George B Waldron was carrying out qualitative research for Mahins Advertising Agency. In 1919, the first book on commercial research was published, Commercial Research: An Outline of Working Principles by Professor C.S. Duncan of the University of Chicago.

Adequate knowledge of consumer preferences was a key to survival in the face of increasingly competitive markets. By the 1920s, advertising agencies, such as J Walter Thompson (JWT), were conducting research on the how and why consumers used brands, so that they could recommend appropriate advertising copy to manufacturers.

The advent of commercial radio in the 1920s, and television in the 1940s, led a number of market research companies to develop the means to measure audience size and audience composition. In 1923, Arthur Nielsen founded market research company, A C Nielsen and over next decade pioneered the measurement of radio audiences. He subsequently applied his methods to the measurement of television audiences. Around the same time, Daniel Starch developed measures for testing advertising copy effectiveness in print media (newspapers and magazines), and these subsequently became known as Starch scores (and are still used today).

During, the 1930s and 1940s, many of the data collection methods, probability sampling methods, survey methods, questionnaire design and key metrics were developed. By the 1930s, Ernest Dichter was pioneering the focus group method of qualitative research. For this, he is often described as the 'father of market research.' Dichter applied his methods on campaigns for major brands including Chrysler, Exxon/Esso where he used methods from psychology and cultural anthropology to gain consumer insights. These methods eventually lead to the development of motivational research. Marketing historians refer to this period as the "Foundation Age" of market research.

By the 1930s, the first courses on marketing research were taught in universities and colleges. The text-book, Market Research and Analysis by Lyndon O. Brown (1937) became one of the popular textbooks during this period. As the number of trained research professionals proliferated throughout the second half of the 20th-century, the techniques and methods used in marketing research became increasingly sophisticated. Marketers, such as Paul Green, were instrumental in developing techniques such as conjoint analysis and multidimensional scaling, both of which are used in positioning maps, market segmentation, choice analysis and other marketing applications.

Web analytics were born out of the need to track the behavior of site visitors and, as the popularity of e-commerce and web advertising grew, businesses demanded details on the information created by new practices in web data collection, such as click-through and exit rates. As the Internet boomed, websites became larger and more complex and the possibility of two-way communication between businesses and their consumers became a reality. Provided with the capacity to interact with online customers, Researchers were able to collect large amounts of data that were previously unavailable, further propelling the marketing research industry.

In the new millennium, as the Internet continued to develop and websites became more interactive, data collection and analysis became more commonplace for those marketing research firms whose clients had a web presence. With the explosive growth of the online marketplace came new competition for companies; no longer were businesses merely competing with the shop down the road — competition was now represented by a global force. Retail outlets were appearing online and the previous need for bricks-and-mortar stores was diminishing at a greater pace than online competition was growing.With so many online channels for consumers to make purchases, companies needed newer and more compelling methods, in combination with messages that resonated more effectively, to capture the attention of the average consumer.

Having access to web data did not automatically provide companies with the rationale behind the behavior of users visiting their sites, which provoked the marketing research industry to develop new and better ways of tracking, collecting and interpreting information. This led to the development of various tools like online focus groups and pop-up or website intercept surveys. These types of services allowed companies to dig deeper into the motivations of consumers, augmenting their insights and utilizing this data to drive market share.

As information around the world became more accessible, increased competition led companies to demand more of market researchers. It was no longer sufficient to follow trends in web behavior or track sales data; companies now needed access to consumer behavior throughout the entire purchase process.This meant the Marketing Research Industry, again, needed to adapt to the rapidly changing needs of the marketplace, and to the demands of companies looking for a competitive edge.

Today, marketing research has adapted to innovations in technology and the corresponding ease with which information is available. B2B and B2C companies are working hard to stay competitive and they now demand both quantitative ("What") and qualitative ("Why?") marketing research in order to better understand their target audience and the motivations behind customer behaviors.

This demand is driving marketing researchers to develop new platforms for interactive, two-way communication between their firms and consumers. Mobile devices such as Smart Phones are the best example of an emerging platform that enables businesses to connect with their customers throughout the entire buying process.

As personal mobile devices become more capable and widespread, the marketing research industry will look to further capitalize on this trend. Mobile devices present the perfect channel for research firms to retrieve immediate impressions from buyers and to provide their clients with a holistic view of the consumers within their target markets, and beyond. Now, more than ever, innovation is the key to success for Marketing Researchers. Marketing Research Clients are beginning to demand highly personalized and specifically-focused products from the marketing research firms; big data is great for identifying general market segments, but is less capable of identifying key factors of niche markets, which now defines the competitive edge companies are looking for in this mobile-digital age.

Characteristics

First, marketing research is systematic. Thus systematic planning is required at all the stages of the marketing research process. The procedures followed at each stage are methodologically sound, well documented, and, as much as possible, planned in advance. Marketing research uses the scientific method in that data are collected and analyzed to test prior notions or hypotheses. Experts in marketing research have shown that studies featuring multiple and often competing hypotheses yield more meaningful results than those featuring only one dominant hypothesis.

Marketing research is objective. It attempts to provide accurate information that reflects a true state of affairs. It should be conducted impartially. While research is always influenced by the researcher's research philosophy, it should be free from the personal or political biases of the researcher or the management. Research which is motivated by personal or political gain involves a breach of professional standards. Such research is deliberately biased so as to result in predetermined findings. The objective nature of marketing research underscores the importance of ethical considerations. Also, researchers should always be objective with regard to the selection of information to be featured in reference texts because such literature should offer a comprehensive view on marketing. Research has shown, however, that many marketing textbooks do not feature important principles in marketing research.

Related business research

Other forms of business research include:

- Market research is broader in scope and examines all aspects of a business environment. It asks questions about competitors, market structure, government regulations, economic trends, technological advances, and numerous other factors that make up the business environment (see environmental scanning). Sometimes the term refers more particularly to the financial analysis of companies, industries, or sectors. In this case, financial analysts usually carry out the research and provide the results to investment advisors and potential investors.
- Product research — This looks at what products can be produced with available technology, and what new product innovations near-future technology can develop (see new product development).

- Advertising research – is a specialized form of marketing research conducted to improve the efficacy of advertising. Copy testing, also known as "pre-testing," is a form of customized research that predicts in-market performance of an ad before it airs, by analyzing audience levels of attention, brand linkage, motivation, entertainment, and communication, as well as breaking down the ad's flow of attention and flow of emotion. Pre-testing is also used on ads still in rough (ripomatic or animatic) form. (Young, p. 213)

Classification

Organizations engage in marketing research for two reasons: firstly, to identify and, secondly, to solve marketing problems. This distinction serves as a basis for classifying marketing research into problem identification research and problem solving research.

Problem identification research is undertaken to help identify problems which are, perhaps, not apparent on the surface and yet exist or are likely to arise in the future like company image, market characteristics, sales analysis, short-range forecasting, long range forecasting, and business trends research. Research of this type provides information about the marketing environment and helps diagnose a problem. For example, the findings of problem solving research are used in making decisions which will solve specific marketing problems.

The Stanford Research Institute, on the other hand, conducts an annual survey of consumers that is used to classify persons into homogeneous groups for segmentation purposes. The National Purchase Diary panel (NPD) maintains the largest diary panel in the United States.

Standardized services are research studies conducted for different client firms but in a standard way. For example, procedures for measuring advertising effectiveness have been standardized so that the results can be compared across studies and evaluative norms can be established. The Starch Readership Survey is the most widely used service for evaluating print advertisements; another well-known service is the Gallup and Robinson Magazine Impact Studies. These services are also sold on a syndicated basis.

- Customized services offer a wide variety of marketing research services customized to suit a client's specific needs. Each marketing research project is treated uniquely.
- Limited-service suppliers specialize in one or a few phases of the marketing research project. Services offered by such suppliers are classified as field services, coding and data entry, data analysis, analytical services, and branded products. Field services collect data through the internet, traditional mail, in-person, or telephone interviewing, and firms that specialize in interviewing are called field service organizations. These organizations may

range from small proprietary organizations which operate locally to large multinational organizations with WATS line interviewing facilities. Some organizations maintain extensive interviewing facilities across the country for interviewing shoppers in malls.

- Coding and data entry services include editing completed questionnaires, developing a coding scheme, and transcribing the data on to diskettes or magnetic tapes for input into the computer. NRC Data Systems provides such services.
- Analytical services include designing and pretesting questionnaires, determining the best means of collecting data, designing sampling plans, and other aspects of the research design. Some complex marketing research projects require knowledge of sophisticated procedures, including specialized experimental designs, and analytical techniques such as conjoint analysis and multidimensional scaling. This kind of expertise can be obtained from firms and consultants specializing in analytical services.
- Data analysis services are offered by firms, also known as tab houses, that specialize in computer analysis of quantitative data such as those obtained in large surveys. Initially most data analysis firms supplied only tabulations (frequency counts) and cross tabulations (frequency counts that describe two or more variables simultaneously). With the proliferation of software, many firms now have the capability to analyze their own data, but, data analysis firms are still in demand.
- Branded marketing research products and services are specialized data collection and analysis procedures developed to address specific types of marketing research problems. These procedures are patented, given brand names, and marketed like any other branded product.

Types

Marketing research techniques come in many forms, including:

- Ad Tracking – periodic or continuous in-market research to monitor a brand's performance using measures such as brand awareness, brand preference, and product usage. (Young, 2005)
- Advertising Research – used to predict copy testing or track the efficacy of advertisements for any medium, measured by the ad's ability to get attention (measured with AttentionTracking), communicate the message, build the brand's image, and motivate the consumer to purchase the product or service. (Young, 2005)
- Brand awareness research — the extent to which consumers can recall or recognize a brand name or product name

- Brand association research — what do consumers associate with the brand?
- Brand attribute research — what are the key traits that describe the brand promise?
- Brand name testing – what do consumers feel about the names of the products?
- Buyer decision making process— to determine what motivates people to buy and what decision-making process they use; over the last decade, Neuromarketing emerged from the convergence of neuroscience and marketing, aiming to understand consumer decision making process
- Commercial eye tracking research — examine advertisements, package designs, websites, etc. by analyzing visual behavior of the consumer
- Concept testing – to test the acceptance of a concept by target consumers
- Coolhunting (also known as trendspotting) – to make observations and predictions in changes of new or existing cultural trends in areas such as fashion, music, films, television, youth culture and lifestyle
- Copy testing – predicts in-market performance of an ad before it airs by analyzing audience levels of attention, brand linkage, motivation, entertainment, and communication, as well as breaking down the ad's flow of attention and flow of emotion. (Young, p 213)
- Customer satisfaction research – quantitative or qualitative studies that yields an understanding of a customer's satisfaction with a transaction
- Demand estimation — to determine the approximate level of demand for the product
- Distribution channel audits — to assess distributors' and retailers' attitudes toward a product, brand, or company
- Internet strategic intelligence — searching for customer opinions in the Internet: chats, forums, web pages, blogs... where people express freely about their experiences with products, becoming strong opinion formers.
- Marketing effectiveness and analytics — Building models and measuring results to determine the effectiveness of individual marketing activities.
- Mystery consumer or mystery shopping – An employee or representative of the market research firm anonymously contacts a salesperson and indicates he or she is shopping for a product. The shopper then records the entire experience. This method is often used for quality control or for researching competitors' products.
- Positioning research — how does the target market see the brand relative to competitors? – what does the brand stand for?

- Price elasticity testing — to determine how sensitive customers are to price changes
- Sales forecasting — to determine the expected level of sales given the level of demand. With respect to other factors like Advertising expenditure, sales promotion etc.
- Segmentation research – to determine the demographic, psychographic, cultural, and behavioral characteristics of potential buyers
- Online panel – a group of individual who accepted to respond to marketing research online
- Store audit — to measure the sales of a product or product line at a statistically selected store sample in order to determine market share, or to determine whether a retail store provides adequate service
- Test marketing — a small-scale product launch used to determine the likely acceptance of the product when it is introduced into a wider market
- Viral Marketing Research – refers to marketing research designed to estimate the probability that specific communications will be transmitted throughout an individual's Social Network. Estimates of Social Networking Potential (SNP) are combined with estimates of selling effectiveness to estimate ROI on specific combinations of messages and media.

All of these forms of marketing research can be classified as either problem-identification research or as problem-solving research.

There are two main sources of data — primary and secondary. Primary research is conducted from scratch. It is original and collected to solve the problem in hand. Secondary research already exists since it has been collected for other purposes. It is conducted on data published previously and usually by someone else. Secondary research costs far less than primary research, but seldom comes in a form that exactly meets the needs of the researcher.

A similar distinction exists between exploratory research and conclusive research. Exploratory research provides insights into and comprehension of an issue or situation. It should draw definitive conclusions only with extreme caution. Conclusive research draws conclusions: the results of the study can be generalized to the whole population.

Exploratory research is conducted to explore a problem to get some basic idea about the solution at the preliminary stages of research. It may serve as the input to conclusive research. Exploratory research information is collected by focus group interviews, reviewing literature or books, discussing with experts, etc. This is unstructured and qualitative in nature. If a secondary source of data is unable to serve the purpose, a convenience sample of small size can be collected. Conclusive research is conducted to draw some conclusion about the problem. It is essentially, structured and quantitative research, and the output of this research is the input to management information systems (MIS).

Exploratory research is also conducted to simplify the findings of the conclusive or descriptive research, if the findings are very hard to interpret for the marketing managers.

Methods

Methodologically, marketing research uses the following types of research designs:

Based on Questioning

- Qualitative marketing research – generally used for exploratory purposes — small number of respondents — not generalizable to the whole population — statistical significance and confidence not calculated — examples include focus groups, in-depth interviews, and projective techniques
- Quantitative marketing research – generally used to draw conclusions — tests a specific hypothesis – uses random sampling techniques so as to infer from the sample to the population — involves a large number of respondents — examples include surveys and questionnaires. Techniques include choice modelling, maximum difference preference scaling, and covariance analysis.

Based on observations

- Ethnographic studies — by nature qualitative, the researcher observes social phenomena in their natural setting — observations can occur cross-sectionally (observations made at one time) or longitudinally (observations occur over several time-periods) – examples include product-use analysis and computer cookie traces. See also Ethnography and Observational techniques.
- Experimental techniques – by nature quantitative, the researcher creates a quasi-artificial environment to try to control spurious factors, then manipulates at least one of the variables — examples include purchase laboratories and test markets.

Researchers often use more than one research design. They may start with secondary research to get background information, then conduct a focus group (qualitative research design) to explore the issues. Finally they might do a full nationwide survey (quantitative research design) in order to devise specific recommendations for the client.

Business to Business

Business to business (B2B) research is inevitably more complicated than consumer research. The researchers need to know what type of multi-faceted approach will answer the objectives, since seldom is it possible to find the answers using just one method. Finding the right respondents is crucial in B2B research since they are often busy, and may not want to participate. Encouraging them to "open up" is yet another skill required of the B2B researcher. Last, but not least, most business research leads to strategic decisions and this means that the business researcher must have expertise in developing strategies that are strongly rooted in the research findings and acceptable to the client.

There are four key factors that make B2B market research special and different from consumer markets:

- The decision making unit is far more complex in B2B markets than in consumer markets.
- B2B products and their applications are more complex than consumer products.
- B2B marketers address a much smaller number of customers who are very much larger in their consumption of products than is the case in consumer markets.
- Personal relationships are of critical importance in B2B markets.

Marketing research does not only occur in huge corporations with many employees and a large budget. Marketing information can be derived by observing the environment of their location and the competitions location. Small scale surveys and focus groups are low cost ways to gather information from potential and existing customers. Most secondary data (statistics, demographics, etc.) is available to the public in libraries or on the internet and can be easily accessed by a small business owner.

Below are some steps that could be done by SME (Small Medium Enterprise) to analyze the market:

1. Provide secondary and or primary data (if necessary);
2. Analyze Macro & Micro Economic data (e.g. Supply & Demand, GDP, Price change, Economic growth, Sales by sector/industries, interest rate, number of investment/ divestment, I/O, CPI, Social analysis, etc.);
3. Implement the marketing mix concept, which is consist of: Place, Price, Product, Promotion, People, Process, Physical Evidence and also Political & social situation to analyze global market situation);
4. Analyze market trends, growth, market size, market share, market competition (e.g. SWOT analysis, B/C Analysis, channel mapping identities of key channels, drivers of customers loyalty and satisfaction, brand percep tion, satisfaction levels, current competitor-channel relationship analysis, etc.), etc.;
5. Determine market segment, market target, market forecast and market position;

6. Formulating market strategy & also investigating the possibility of partnership/ collaboration (e.g. Profiling & SWOT analysis of potential partners, evaluating business partnership.)
7. Combine those analysis with the SME's business plan/ business model analysis (e.g. Business description, Business process, Business strategy, Revenue model, Business expansion, Return of Investment, Financial analysis (Company History, Financial assumption, Cost/Benefit Analysis, Projected profit & Loss, Cash flow, Balance sheet & business Ratio, etc.).

INTERNATIONAL PLAN

International Marketing Research follows the same path as domestic research, but there are a few more problems that may arise. Customers in international markets may have very different customs, cultures, and expectations from the same company. In this case, Marketing Research relies more on primary data rather than secondary information. Gathering the primary data can be hindered by language, literacy and access to technology. Basic Cultural and Market intelligence information will be needed to maximize the research effectiveness. Some of the steps that would help overcoming barriers include:

1. Collect secondary information on the country under study from reliable international source e.g. WHO and IMF
2. Collect secondary information on the product/service under study from available sources
3. Collect secondary information on product manufacturers and service providers under study in relevant country
4. Collect secondary information on culture and common business practices
5. Ask questions to get better understanding of reasons behind any recommendations for a specific methodology

Common Terms

Market research techniques resemble those used in political polling and social science research. Meta-analysis (also called the Schmidt-Hunter technique) refers to a statistical method of combining data from multiple studies or from several types of studies. Conceptualization means the process of converting vague mental images into definable concepts. Operationalization is the process of converting concepts into specific observable behaviors that a researcher can measure. Precision refers to the exactness of any given measure. Reliability refers to the likelihood that a given operationalized construct will yield the same results if re-measured. Validity refers to the extent to which a measure provides data that captures the meaning of the operationalized construct as defined in the study. It asks, "Are we measuring what we intended to measure?"

- Applied research sets out to prove a specific hypothesis of value to the clients paying for the research. For example, a cigarette company might commission research that attempts to show that cigarettes are good for one's health. Many researchers have ethical misgivings about doing applied research.
- Sugging (from SUG, for "selling under the guise" of market research) forms a sales technique in which sales people pretend to conduct marketing research, but with the real purpose of obtaining buyer motivation and buyer decision-making information to be used in a subsequent sales call.
- Frugging comprises the practice of soliciting funds under the pretense of being a research organization.

Careers

Some of the positions available in marketing research include vice president of marketing research, research director, assistant director of research, project manager, field work director, statistician/data processing specialist, senior analyst, analyst, junior analyst and operational supervisor.

The most common entry-level position in marketing research for people with bachelor's degrees (e.g., BBA) is as operational supervisor. These people are responsible for supervising a well-defined set of operations, including field work, data editing, and coding, and may be involved in programming and data analysis. Another entry-level position for BBAs is assistant project manager. An assistant project manager will learn and assist in questionnaire design, review field instructions, and monitor timing and costs of studies. In the marketing research industry, however, there is a growing preference for people with master's degrees. Those with MBA or equivalent degrees are likely to be employed as project managers.

A small number of business schools also offer a more specialized Master of Marketing Research (MMR) degree. An MMR typically prepares students for a wide range of research methodologies and focuses on learning both in the classroom and the field.

The typical entry-level position in a business firm would be junior research analyst (for BBAs) or research analyst (for MBAs or MMRs). The junior analyst and the research analyst learn about the particular industry and receive training from a senior staff member, usually the marketing research manager. The junior analyst position includes a training program to prepare individuals for the responsibilities of a research analyst, including coordinating with the marketing department and sales force to develop goals for product exposure. The research analyst responsibilities include checking all data for accuracy, comparing and contrasting new research with established norms, and analyzing primary and secondary data for the purpose of market forecasting.

As these job titles indicate, people with a variety of backgrounds and skills are needed in marketing research. Technical specialists such as statisticians obviously need strong backgrounds in statistics and data analysis. Other positions, such as research director, call for managing the work of others and require more general skills. To prepare for a career in marketing research, students usually:

- Take all the marketing courses.
- Take courses in statistics and quantitative methods.
- Acquire computer skills.
- Take courses in psychology and consumer behavior.
- Acquire effective written and verbal communication skills.
- Think creatively.

Corporate Hierarchy

1. Vice-President of Marketing Research: This is the senior position in marketing research. The VP is responsible for the entire marketing research operation of the company and serves on the top management team. Sets the objectives and goals of the marketing research department.
2. Research Director: Also a senior position, the director has the overall responsibility for the development and execution of all the marketing research projects.
3. Assistant Director of Research: Serves as an administrative assistant to the director and supervises some of the other marketing research staff members.
4. (Senior) Project Manager: Has overall responsibility for design, implementation, and management of research projects.
5. Statistician/Data Processing Specialist: Serves as an expert on theory and application of statistical techniques. Responsibilities include experimental design, data processing, and analysis.
6. Senior Analyst: Participates in the development of projects and directs the operational execution of the assigned projects. Works closely with the analyst, junior analyst, and other personnel in developing the research design and data collection. Prepares the final report. The primary responsibility for meeting time and cost constraints rests with the senior analyst.
7. Analyst: Handles the details involved in executing the project. Designs and pretests the questionnaires and conducts a preliminary analysis of the data.
8. Junior Analyst: Handles routine assignments such as secondary data analysis, editing and coding of questionnaires, and simple statistical analysis.
9. Field Work Director: Responsible for the selection, training, supervision, and evaluation of interviewers and other field workers.

The marketing research process is a six-step process involving the definition of the problem being studied upon, determining what approach to take, formulation of research design, field work entailed, data preparation and analysis, and the generation of reports, how to present these reports, and overall, how the task can be accomplished.

The first stage in a marketing research project is to define the problem. In defining the problem, the researcher should take into account the purpose of the study, relevant background information and all necessary data, and how the information gathered will be used in decision making. Problem definition involves discussion with the decision makers, interviews with industry experts, analysis of secondary data, and, perhaps, some qualitative research, such as focus groups. Once the problem has been precisely defined, the research can be designed and conducted properly.

Development of an approach to the problem is the second step. This includes formulating an objective or theoretical framework, constructing analytical models, generating research questions, hypotheses, and identifying characteristics or factors that can influence the research design. This process is guided by discussions with management and industry experts, case studies and simulations, analysis of secondary data, qualitative research and pragmatic considerations.

The third step involves the formulation of the research design which is the framework or blueprint for conducting the marketing research project. It details the procedures necessary in obtaining the required information, and its purpose is to design a study that will test the hypotheses of interest, determine possible answers to the research questions, and provide the information necessary for decision making. Conducting exploratory research, precisely defining the variables, and designing appropriate scales to measure them are also components of the research design. The issue on how the data should be obtained from the respondents must be addressed. It is also necessary to design a questionnaire and a sampling plan to select respondents for the study.

Formulating the research design involves the following steps:

1. Secondary data analysis
2. Qualitative research
3. Methods of collecting quantitative data (survey, observation, and experimentation)
4. Definition of the information needed
5. Measurement and scaling procedures
6. Questionnaire design
7. Sampling process and sample size
8. Plan of data analysis

Fourth is data collection which involves manpower/staff members who operate either in the field, as in the case of personal interviewing (in-home, mall intercept, or computer-assisted personal interviewing), from an office by telephone (telephone or computer-assisted telephone interviewing), or through mail (traditional mail and mail panel surveys with pre-recruited households). Proper selection, training, supervision, and evaluation of staff members helps minimize data-collection errors.

Data preparation and analysis is the fifth step and includes the editing, coding, transcription, and verification of data. Each questionnaire or observation form is inspected, or edited, and, if necessary, corrected. Number or letter codes are assigned to represent each response to each question in the questionnaire. The data from the questionnaires are transcribed or key-punched on to magnetic tapes, or disks or inputted directly into the computer. Verification ensures that the data from the original questionnaires have been accurately transcribed.

Analyzed data gives meaning to the information that have been collected. Univariate techniques are used for analyzing data when there is a single measurement of each element or unit in the sample, or, if there are several measurements of each element, each RCH variable is analyzed in isolation. On the other hand, multivariate techniques are used for analyzing data when there are two or more measurements on each element and the variables are analyzed simultaneously.

The last stage is the report preparation and presentation. The entire project should be documented in a written report and the results and major findings must be presented. The findings must be in a comprehensible format so that they can be readily used in the decision making process. In addition, an oral presentation should be made to management using tables, figures, and graphs to enhance clarity and impact.

For these reasons, interviews with experts are more useful in conducting marketing research for industrial firms and for products of a technical nature, where it is relatively easy to identify and approach the experts. This method is also helpful in situations where little information is available from other sources, as in the case of radically new products.

Primary Data Vs. Secondary Data

Primary data is sourced by the researcher for the specific purpose of addressing the research problem. On the other hand, secondary data is collected for some purpose other than the problem at hand. This data includes information made available by business and government sources, commercial marketing research firms, and computerized databases. Secondary data is an economical and quick source of background information.

Qualitative Research

Information, industry experts, and secondary data may not be sufficient to define the research problem. Sometimes qualitative research must be undertaken to gain a qualitative understanding of the problem and its underlying factors. Qualitative research is unstructured, exploratory in nature, based on small samples, and may utilize popular qualitative techniques such as focus groups (group interviews), word association (asking respondents to indicate their first responses to stimulus words), and depth interviews (one-on-one interviews which probe the respondents' thoughts in detail). Other exploratory research techniques, such as pilot surveys with small samples of respondents, may also be undertaken.

6

Innovation Policy and the Market for Vaccines

When it comes to vaccines, India has worked diligently to make a name for itself. It is the world's largest supplier of vaccines, producing 62% of global demand. Since 2012 India's pharmaceutical industry market value has been growing significantly. The vaccine storage temperature and cold chain logistics play a large role in how India is able to safely deliver life-saving vaccines all across the globe.

There have been great strides around the world in the development of vaccines in the last 60 years. Currently, there are vaccines to prevent 20 life-threatening diseases. Through the help of the World Health Organization (WHO), there is a global outreach to bring vaccines to poorer countries where preventative healthcare isn't as readily accessible. By reaching these underserved areas, it helps prevent infectious disease outbreaks on a global level.

The establishment of the Universal Immunisation Programme (UIP), first adopted in 1978 and adapted several times over the years, developed a vaccine protocol for children, with a recommended schedule for high life-threatening, extremely high life-threatening, moderate life-threatening, and low life-threatening potential diseases. With the establishment of the National Rural Health Mission in 2005, the community outreach for administering vaccines to the rural and underserved areas has improved.

According to McKinsey, in 2012, India's pharmaceutical market share was less than desirable at $ 500 million. At that time, nearly two million Indian lives were lost per year, most of which were children due to vaccine-preventable deaths. India saw an opportunity to right a wrong for its citizens and improve business opportunities throughout the country.

India and the Vaccine Marketplace

India is the largest manufacturing region for vaccines worldwide. Currently, two-thirds of its production is exported, while one-third is used domestically, with the UIP helping to distribute the vaccines countrywide. While production has grown significantly, the Indian pharmaceutical industry is expected to climb to 65 billion USD by 2024.

Cost Efficiency of India Vaccines

India's low cost of production, research and development contribute to the country's cost efficiency of not only vaccines but all their pharmaceuticals. According to investindia.gov, producing pharmaceuticals in India is 33% less costly than that of western markets. Their ability to keep costs down directly correlates to their high export numbers making vaccines obtainable for even the poorest of populations.

Generic Drug Industry

India is the world's largest manufacturing region and exporter of generic medicines. It contributes 60,000 generic brands within 60 therapeutic categories, exporting approximately two-thirds of all its supplies to countries worldwide.

Their generic drug industry is being threatened due to strict regulations being placed on exports of medicinal products. In August of 2020, President Trump signed an executive order disallowing drug imports, both as active ingredients and formulations. While France and Germany appear to be heading in the same direction. For now, India remains the leading manufacturing market in the generic drug industry.

India vs. China

The world has watched as India thrived in the world of pharmaceuticals, but China has not only taken note but also decided they need a piece of the market. Beijing's "Made in China 2025" has included pharmaceuticals as part of its targeted campaign.

India's claim to fame is its ability to manufacture and export affordable medications across the globe, particularly to the most impoverished countries.

Fortunately, it is currently believed that China will maintain its efforts to establish itself as a formulator of pharmaceuticals leaving India to rule the generic medication field. But with both vying for raw products, there is some concern that it might drive up the cost of production, edging out India's lead on the affordable healthcare market.

Why Temperature-Controlled Shipping is Necessary?

The vaccine storage temperature must be closely managed and controlled to maintain the vaccine's efficacy. Some vaccines are more susceptible to heat, such as the measles and DTP vaccines, and others are more cold-sensitive such as Heb B and Hib (in liquid form). Once its viability is lost, it cannot be restored.

Since most of India's vaccines are exported to other countries, maintaining a correct vaccine storage temperature during transport is of the highest importance. Vaccines have a short shelf-life, so shipping by air is a preferred means of transport for many vaccine manufacturers. To ensure that shipments arrive safely and intact, air freight supply chain stakeholders follow strict vaccine storage and handling requirements as defined by the shipper/manufacturer in the cold chain process. Vaccines' active ingredients may lose potency or even be destroyed if the temperature is not maintained between (2?–8?), or -20°C for some products, so the vaccine cold or frozen storage and transport system is essential across the supply chain.

What is the Role of the Cold Chain Logistics Stakeholders?

Stakeholders have the responsibility of identifying and mitigating the risk of damage to vaccine shipments within the cold chain logistics. They should each make sure that the vaccine storage temperature is well maintained at every step of the way while the consignment is in their area of responsibility. This applies to all critical control points and stakeholders in the process from manufacturing to patient, including all important air freight supply chain stakeholders like forwarders, ground handling agents, airlines, warehouse operators and trucking vendors.

Cold Chain Logistics

Maintaining strict vaccine storage, handling and transport requirements for cold chain logistics is how vaccines can be shipped effectively worldwide. Even though the roles may differ, the same quality and risk management principles must be followed no matter where a stakeholder may be in the cold chain supply chain. Stakeholders involved should always follow, good storage practices (GSP), and good and distribution practice (GDP).

Manufacturers

The vaccine supply chain begins with the manufacturers. It is their responsibility to properly prepare the vaccines for shipment. This not only includes appropriately packaging and labeling of vaccine shipments for cold or frozen storage, it also means ensuring all documentation is in order so there are no issues with customs or foreign state requirements, allowing the vaccines to arrive in a timely manner

Freight Forwarders

The freight forwarders are responsible for selecting and engaging only those subcontractors that are approved and have a required knowledge and quality and risk management systems in place for safe handling and transport of vaccines.

Vendors offering temperature-controlled road transport meet vaccine storage and handling requirements by carrying the vaccine cold storage at predefined and communicated temperature range and set points to ensure product safety and efficacy. The qualified temperature-controlled trucks are an essential part of the cold chain logistics enabling vaccines to safely move between the supply chain points.

Airlines

It is the airlines who will do most of the worldwide shipping. Shipping by airallows vaccines to reach distant destinations in a timely manner. This is crucial since the shelf-life of many vaccines is short-lived. Airlines must adhere to the vaccine storage and handling requirements before, during, and after the flight between transfers with the freight forwarders.

Once received from the freight forwarders, the vaccines must be stored in qualified temperature-controlled storage premises at the airlines' or ground handling service providers facilities while waiting for aircraft loading to commence. During this time, the shipment will be cross-checked for all relevant safety requirements, such as checking appropriate labels, checking the air waybill, temperature-controlled instructions and overall condition of the shipment before making it ready for carriage. This is managed by using IATA mandatory check list for time and temperature sensitive products. Considering the process duration, exposure to external temperature conditions needs to be minimized and wherever possible, maintained at the predefined temperature range.

GOALS OF VACCINATION POLICIES

Immunity and herd immunity

Vaccination policies aim to produce immunity to preventable diseases. Besides individual protection from getting ill, some vaccination policies also aim to provide the community as a whole with herd immunity. Herd immunity refers to the idea that the pathogen will have trouble spreading when a significant part of the population has immunity against it. This protects those unable to get the vaccine due to medical conditions, such as immune disorders.

Vaccine-preventable diseases remain the most common cause of childhood mortality with an estimated three million deaths each year. Each year, vaccination prevents between two and three million deaths worldwide, across all age groups, from diphtheria, tetanus, pertussis and measles.

Eradication of disease

With some vaccines, a goal of vaccination policies is to eradicate the disease – make it disappear from Earth altogether. The World Health Organization coordinated the effort to eradicate smallpox globally through vaccination, the last naturally occurring case of smallpox was in Somalia in 1977. Endemic measles, mumps and rubella have been eliminated through vaccination in Finland. The WHO has targeted polio for eradication by the year 2018.

Individual versus group goals

Rational individuals will attempt to minimize the risk of illness, and will seek vaccination for themselves or their children if they perceive a high threat of disease and a low risk to vaccination. However, if a vaccination program successfully reduces the disease threat, it may reduce the perceived risk of disease enough so that an individual's optimal strategy is to encourage everyone but their family to be vaccinated, or (more generally) to refuse vaccination once vaccination rates reach a certain level, even if this level is below that optimal for the community. For example, a 2003 study found that a bioterrorist attack using smallpox would result in conditions where voluntary vaccination would be unlikely to reach the optimum level for the U.S. as a whole, and a 2007 study found that severe influenza epidemics cannot be prevented by voluntary vaccination without offering certain incentives. Governments often allow exemptions to mandatory vaccinations for religious or philosophical reasons, but decreased rates of vaccination may cause loss of herd immunity, substantially increasing risks even to vaccinated individuals. However, mandatory vaccination policies raise ethical issues regarding parental rights and informed consent.

Compulsory vaccination

At various times governments and other institutions have established policies requiring vaccination, with the aim of reducing the risk of disease. For example, an 1853 law required universal vaccination against smallpox in England and Wales, with fines levied on people who did not comply. In the United States, the Supreme Court ruled in Jacobson v. Massachusetts (1905) that states have the authority to require vaccination against smallpox during a smallpox epidemic. All 50 U.S states require that children be vaccinated in order to attend school; although 47 states provide exemptions based on religious or philosophical beliefs. A few other countries also follow this practice. Compulsory vaccination greatly reduces infection rates for associated diseases. These policies stirred resistance from a variety of groups, collectively called anti-vaccinationists, who objected on ethical, political, medical safety, religious, and other grounds. Common objections included the argument that governments should not infringe on an individual's freedom to make medical decisions for themselves or their children, or claims that proposed vaccinations were dangerous. Many modern vaccination policies allow exemptions for people with compromised immune systems, allergies to vaccination components, or strongly held objections. It has also been argued that for vaccination to effectively prevent disease, there must not only be available vaccines and a population willing to immunize, but also sufficient ability to decline vaccination on grounds of personal belief.

In 1904 in the city of Rio de Janeiro, Brazil, following an urban renewal program that displaced many poor, a government program of mandatory smallpox vaccination triggered theVaccine Revolt, several days of rioting with considerable property damage and a number of deaths.

Compulsory vaccination is a difficult policy issue, requiring authorities to balance public health with individual liberty:

"Vaccination is unique among de facto mandatory requirements in the modern era, requiring individuals to accept the injection of a medicine or medicinal agent into their bodies, and it has provoked a spirited opposition. This opposition began with the first vaccinations, has not ceased, and probably never will. From this realisation arises a difficult issue: how should the mainstream medical authorities approach the anti-vaccination movement? A passive reaction could be construed as endangering the health of society, whereas a heavy-handed approach can threaten the values of individual liberty and freedom of expression that we cherish."

Investigation of different types of vaccination policy finds strong evidence that standing orders and allowing healthcare workers without prescription authority (such as nurses) to administer vaccines in defined circumstances increases vaccination rates, and sufficient evidence that requiring vaccinations before attending child care and school does so. but insufficient evidence to assess effectiveness of requiring vaccinations as a condition for hospital and other healthcare jobs.

Many countries, including Canada, Germany, Japan, and the United States have specific requirements for reporting vaccine-related adverse effects, while other countries including Australia, France, and the United Kingdom include vaccines under their general requirements for reporting injuries associated with medical treatments. A number of countries have both compulsory vaccination and national programs for the compensation of injuries alleged to have been caused by a vaccination.

Children's rights

Medical ethicist Arthur Caplan argues that children have a right to the best available medical care, including vaccines, regardless of parental feelings toward vaccines, saying "Arguments about medical freedom and choice are at odds with the human and constitutional rights of children. When parents won't protect them, governments must."

To prevent the spread of disease by unvaccinated individuals, some schools and doctors' surgeries have prohibited unvaccinated children from being enrolled, even where not required by law. Refusal of doctors to treat unvaccinated children may cause harm to both the child and public health, and may be considered unethical, if the parents are unable to find another healthcare provider for the child. Opinion on this is divided, with the largest professional association, the American Academy of Pediatrics, saying that exclusion of unvaccinated children may be an option under narrowly defined circumstances.

Evaluating vaccination policy

Vaccines as a positive externality

The promotion of high levels of vaccination produces the protective effect of herd immunity as well as positive externalities in society. Vaccinations are public goods, they are both non-rivalrous and non-excludable, and given these traits, individuals may avoid the costs of vaccination by "free-riding" off the benefits of others being vaccinated. The costs and benefits to individuals and society have been studied and critiqued in stable and changing population designs. Other surveys have indicated that free-riding incentives exist in individual decisions, and in a separate study that looked at parental vaccination choice, the study found that parents were less likely to vaccinate their children if their children's friends had already been vaccinated.

Since the first economic analysis of routine childhood immunizations in the United States in 2001 that reported cost savings over the lifetime of children born in 2001, other analyses of the economic costs and potential benefits to individuals and society have since been studied, evaluated, and calculated. In 2014, the American Academy of Pediatrics published a decision analysis that evaluated direct costs (program costs such as vaccine cost, administrative burden, negative vaccine-linked reactions, and transportation time lost to parents to seek health providers for vaccination). The study focused on diphtheria, tetanus, pertussis, Haemophilus influenza type b conjugate, poliovirus, measles/mumps/rubella (MMR), hepatitis B, varicella, 7-valent pneumococcal conjugate, hepatitis A, and rotavirus vaccines, but excluded influenza. Estimated costs and benefits were adjusted to 2009 dollars and projected over time at 3% annual interest rate. Of the theoretical group of 4,261,494 babies beginning in 2009, that had regular immunizations through childhood in accordance with the Advisory Committee on Immunization Practices guidelines "will prevent <"42 000 early deaths and 20 million cases of disease, with net savings of $13.5 billion in direct costs and $68.8 billion in total societal costs, respectively." In the United States, and in other nations, there is an economic incentive and "global value" to invest in preventive vaccination programs, especially in children as a means to prevent early infant and childhood deaths.

International Organizations

In 2006, the World Health Organization and UNICEF created the Global Immunization Vision and Strategy (GIVS). This organization created a ten-year strategy with four main goals:

- to immunize more people against more diseases
- to introduce a range of newly available vaccines and technologies
- to integrate other critical health interventions with immunization
- to manage vaccination programmes within the context of global interdependence

The Global Vaccination Action Plan was created by the World Health Organization and endorsed by the World Health Assembly in 2012. The plan which is set from 2011–2020 is intended to "strengthen routine immunization to meet vaccination coverage targets; accelerate control of vaccine-preventable diseases with polio eradication as the first milestone; introduce new and improved vaccines and spur research and development for the next generation of vaccines and technologies".

Policies and history by country

In December 2018, Argentina enacted a new vaccine policy requiring all persons who are medically able, both adults and children, to be vaccinated against specified diseases. Proof of vaccination is required to attend any level of school, from infancy through adulthood, or obtain a marriage license, or any kind of government ID, including a passport or driver's license. Furthermore, the law requires the government to pay for all aspects of all vaccinations. The law deems vaccination to be a national emergency, and therefore exempts vaccines from internal and customs taxes.

Australia

In an effort to boost vaccination rates in Australia, the Australian government has decided that starting on 1 January 2016, certain benefits (such as the universal 'Family Allowance' welfare payments for parents of children) will no longer be available for conscientious objectors of vaccination; those with medical grounds for not vaccinating will continue to receive such benefits. The policy is supported by a majority of Australian parents as well as the Australian Medical Association (AMA) and Early Childhood Australia. In 2014, about 97 percent of children under 7 years were vaccinated, though the number of conscientious objectors to vaccination has increased by 24,000 to 39,000 over the past decade.

The government began the Immunise Australia Program to increase national immunisation rates. They fund a number of different vaccinations for certain groups of people. The intent is to encourage the most at-risk populations to get vaccinated. The government maintains an immunization schedule.

China

Children get compulsory vaccines under a state-sponsored health programme at hospitals and disease control centres. DPT vaccine has been given to children since the 1970s.Hepatitis B, rabies and influenza vaccines are optional and provided mainly on a commercial basis. Both the Changsheng Bio-Technology Co Ltd and the Wuhan Institute of Biological Products have been fined for selling ineffective vaccines. In December 2018, China enacted new laws imposing strict controls over the production and inspection of aspects of vaccine production from research, development, and testing through production and distribution.

France

Vaccination Schedule 2015

In France, the High Council of Public Health is in charge of proposing vaccine recommendations to the Minister of Health. Each year, immunization recommendations for both the general population and specific groups are published by the Institute of Epidemiology and Surveillance. Since some hospitals are granted additional freedoms, there two key people responsible for vaccine policy within hospitals: the Operational physician (OP), and the Head of the hospital infection and prevention committee (HIPC). Mandatory immunization policies on BCG, diphtheria, tetanus, and poliomyelitis began in the 1950s and policies on Hepatitis B began in 1991. Recommended but not mandatory suggestions on influenza, pertussis, varicella, and measles began in 2000, 2004, 2004, and 2005, respectively. According to the 2013 INPES Peretti-Watel health barometer, between 2005 and 2010, the percentage of French people between 18–75 years old in favor of vaccination dropped from 90% to 60%.

Since 2009, France has recommended meningococcus C vaccination for infants 1–2 years old, with a catch up dosage up to 25 years later. French insurance companies have reimbursed this vaccine since January 2010, at which point coverage levels were 32.3% for children 1–2 years and 21.3% for teenagers 14–16 years old. In 2012, the French government and the Institut de veille sanitaire launched a 5-year national program in order to improve vaccination policy. The program simplified guidelines, facilitated access to vaccination, and invested in vaccine research. In 2014, fueled by rare health-related scandals, mistrust of vaccines became a common topic in the French public debate on health. According to a French radio station, as of 2014, 3 to 5 percent of kids in France were not given the mandatory vaccines. Some families may avoid requirements by finding a doctor willing to forge a vaccination certificate, a solution which numerous French forums confirm. However, the French State considers "vaccine refusal" a form of child abuse. In some instances, parental vaccine refusals may result in criminal trials. France's 2010 creation of the Question Prioritaire Constitutionelle (QPC) allows lower courts to refer constitutional questions to the highest court in the relevant hierarchy. Therefore, criminal trials based on vaccine refusals may be referred to the Cour de Cassation, which will then certify whether the case meets certain criteria. In May 2015, France updated its vaccination policies on diphtheria, tetanus, acellular pertussis, polio, Haemophilus influenzae b infections, and hepatitis B for premature infants. As of 2015, while failure to vaccinate is not necessarily illegal, a parent's right to refuse to vaccinate his or her child is technically a constitutional matter. Additionally, children in France cannot enter schools without proof of vaccination against diphtheria, tetanus, and polio. French Health Minister, Marisol Touraine, finds vaccinations "absolutely fundamental to avoid disease," and has pushed to have both trained pharmacists and doctors administer vaccinations. Most recently, the Prime Minister's 2015–2017 roadmap for the "multi-annual social inclusion and anti-poverty plan" includes free vaccinations in certain public facilities. Vaccinations within the immunization schedule are given for free at immunization services within the public sector. When given in private medical practices, vaccinations are 65% reimbursed.

Germany

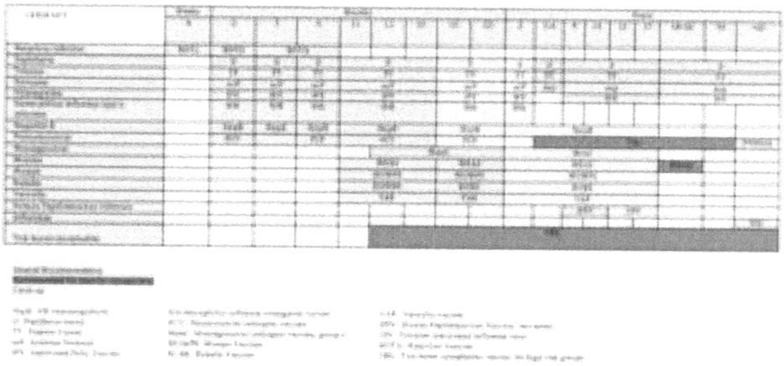

Vaccination Schedule 2015

In Germany, the Standing Committee on Vaccination (STIKO) is the federal commission responsible for recommending an immunization schedule. The Robert Koch Institute in Berlin (RKI) compiles data of immunization status upon the entry of children at school, and measures vaccine coverage of Germany at a national level. Founded in 1972, the STIKO is composed of 12–18 volunteers, appointed members by the Federal Ministry for Health for 3-year terms. Members include experts from many scientific disciplines and public health fields and professionals with extensive experience on vaccination.The independent advisory group meets biannually to address issues pertaining to preventable infectious diseases.Although the STIKO makes recommendations, immunization in Germany is voluntary and there are no official government recommendations. German Federal States typically follow the Standing Vaccination Committee's recommendations minimally, although each state can make recommendations for their geographic jurisdiction that extends beyond the recommended list. In addition to the proposed immunization schedule for children and adults, the STIKO recommends vaccinations for occupational groups, police, travelers, and other at risk groups. Vaccinations recommendations that are issued must be in accordance with the Protection Against Infection Act (Infektionsschutzgesetz), which regulates the prevention of infectious diseases in humans. If a vaccination is recommended because of occupational risks, it must adhere to the Occupational Safety and Health Act involving Biological Agents. Criteria for the recommendation include disease burden, efficacy and effectiveness, safety, feasibility of program implementation, cost-effectiveness evaluation, clinical trial results, and equity in access to the vaccine. In the event of vaccination related injuries, federal states are responsible for monetary compensation. Germany's central government does not finance childhood immunizations, so 90% of vaccines are administered in a private physician's office and paid for through insurance. The other 10% of vaccines are provided by the states in public health clinics, schools, or day care centers by local immunization programs. Physician responsibilities concerning immunization include beginning infancy vaccination, administering booster vaccinations, maintaining medical and vaccination history, and giving information and recommendations concerning vaccines.

Ireland

In the Republic of Ireland, childhood vaccination (up to age 16) requires the consent of the parents. The Department of Health strongly recommend vaccinations.

Italy

As aging populations in Italy bring a rising burden of age-related disease, the Italian vaccination system remains complex.The fact that services and decisions are delivered by 21 separate regional authorities creates many variations in Italian vaccine policy. There is a National committee on immunizations that updates the national recommended immunization schedule, with input from the ministry of health representatives, regional health authorities, national institute of health, and other scientific societies. Regions may add more scheduled vaccinations, but cannot exempt citizens from nationally mandated or recommended ones. For instance, a nationwide plan for eliminating measles and rubella began in 2001.Certain vaccinations in Italy are based on findings from the National Centre for Epidemiology, Surveillance and Health Promotion are also used to determine miscellaneous vaccination mandates.

Childhood vaccinations included in national schedules are guaranteed free of charge for all Italian children and foreign children who live in the country. Estimated insurance coverage for the required three doses of HBV-Hib-IPV vaccines is at least 95% when the child is 2 years old. Later, Influenza is the only nationally necessary vaccine for adults, and is administered by general practitioners. To mitigate some public concerns, Italy currently has a national vaccine injury compensation program. Essentially, those who are ill or damaged by mandatory and recommended vaccinations may receive funding from the government as compensation. One evaluation of vaccine coverage in 2010, which covered the 2008 birth cohort, showed a slight decline in immunization insurance coverage rates of diphtheria, hepatitis B, polio, and tetanus after those specific vaccinations had been made mandatory. However, vaccination levels continued to pass the Italian government's goal of 95% outreach.

Aiming to integrate immunization strategies across the country and equitize access to disease prevention, the Italian Ministry of Health issued the National Immunization Prevention Plan (Piano Nazionale Prevenzione Vaccinale) in 2012. This plan for 2012–2014 introduced an institutional "lifecourse" approach to vaccination to complement the Italian health policy agenda. HPV vaccine coverage increased well, and pneumococcal vaccine and meningococcal C vaccines faced positive public reception. However, both infant vaccine coverage rates and influenza immunization in the elderly have been decreasing. A 2015 government plan in Italy aimed to boost vaccination rates and introduce a series of new vaccines, triggering protests among public health professionals. Partially in response to the statistic that less than 86% of Italian children receive the measles shot, the National Vaccination Plan for 2016–18 (PNPV) increased vaccination requirements. For instance, nationwide varicella shots would be required for newborns. Under this plan, government spending on vaccines would double to €620 million annually, and children could be barred from attending school without proving vaccination. Although these implementations would make Italy a European frontrunner in vaccination, some experts questioned the need for several of the vaccines, and some physicians worried about the potential punishment they may face if they do not comply with the proposed regulations.

There were 5,000 cases of measles in 2017, up from 870 in 2016, 29% of all those in the European Union. The law compelling children to have 10 vaccinations in order to enrol at state schools came into effect in March 2018 but in August 2018 the Five Star Movement pushed legislation through the Italian Senate abolishing it. It did not pass the Chamber of Deputies but parents did not have to provide schools with a doctor's note to show their children have been vaccinated. By November 2018 the government had changed its stance because of the "measles emergency" and decided to uphold the obligation for children up to the age of 16, teachers and health professionals to be vaccinated. A midwife working at a hospital in central Italy was sacked for refusing vaccination.

Latvia

According to a 2011 publication in CMAJ: The notion of "mandatory" in Latvia differs from that of other nations. Latvia appears unique in that it compels health care providers to obtain the signatures of those who decline vaccination. Individuals have the right to refuse a vaccination, but if they do so, health providers have a duty to explain the health consequences.

Vaccines that are not mandatory are not publicly funded, so the cost for those must be borne by parents or employers, she adds. Funded vaccinations include tuberculosis, diphtheria, measles, hepatitis B, human papilloma virus for 12-year-old girls, and tick-borne encephalitis until age 18 in endemic areas and for orphans.

Malaysia

In Malaysia, mass vaccination is practised in public schools. The vaccines may be administered by a school nurse or a team of other medical staff from outside the school. All the children in a given school year are vaccinated as a cohort. For example, children may receive the oral polio vaccine in Year One of primary school (about six or seven years of age), the BCG in Year Six, and the MMR in Form Three of secondary school. Therefore, most people have received their core vaccines by the time they finish secondary school.

Nigeria

In Nigeria, the Expanded Programme on Immunization (EPI), was introduced in 1978 to provide free immunization against polio, measles, diphtheria, whooping cough, tuberculosis, and yellow fever to Nigerian children less than 2 years old. This free immunization can be obtained at any primary health centre in the country. The vaccines are usually administered by a government health care worker. They also conduct routine vaccination visits in schools where all the children in a given school are vaccinated.

Pakistan

Facing numerous minor polio epidemics, the Pakistani government has now ruled that the polio vaccination as mandatory and indisputable. In a statement from Pakistani Police Commissioner Riaz Khan Mehsud "There is no mercy, we have decided to deal with the refusal cases with iron hands. Anyone who refuses [the vaccine] will be sent to jail".

Slovenia

According to a 2011 publication in CMAJ: Slovenia has one of the world's most aggressive and comprehensive vaccination programs. Its program is mandatory for nine designated diseases. Within the first three months of life, infants must be vaccinated for tuberculosis, tetanus, polio, pertussis, and Haemophilus influenza type B. Within 18 months, vaccines are required for measles, mumps and rubella, and finally, before a child starts school, the child must be vaccinated for hepatitis B. While a medical exemption request can be submitted to a committee, such an application for reasons of religion or conscience would not be acceptable. Failure to comply results in a fine and compliance rates top 95%, Kraigher says, adding that for nonmandatory vaccines, such as the one for human papilloma virus, coverage is below 50%.

Mandatory vaccination against measles was introduced in 1968 and since 1978, all children receive two doses of vaccine with a compliance rate of more than 95%. For TBE, the vaccination rate in 2007 was estimated to be 12.4% of the general population in 2007. For comparison, in neighboring Austria, 87% of the population is vaccinated against TBE.

South Africa

The South African Vaccination and Immunisation Centre began in 2003 as an alliance between the South African Department of Health, vaccine industry, academic institutions and other stakeholders. SAIVC works with WHO and the South African National Department of Health to educate, do research, provide technical support, and advocate. They work to increase rates of vaccination in order to improve the nation's health.

Spain

Spain's 19 autonomous communities, consisting of 17 Regions and 2 cities, follow health policies established by the Inter-Territorial Health Council that was formed by the National and Regional Ministries of Health. This Inter-Territorial Council is composed of representatives from each region and meets to discuss health related issues spanning across Spain. The Institute of Health Carlos III (ISCIIII) is a public research institute that manages biomedical research for the advancement of health sciences and disease preventions. The ISCIII may suggest the introduction of new vaccines into Spain's Recommended Health Schedule and is under direct control of the Ministry of Health. Although the Ministry of Health is responsible for the oversight of health care services, the policy of devolution divides responsibilities among local agencies, including health planning and programing, fiscal duties, and direct management of health services. This decentralization proposes difficulties in collecting information at the national level. The Inter-Territorial Council's Commission on Public Health works to establish health care policies according to recommendations by technical working groups via letters, meetings, and conferences. The Technical Working Group on Vaccines review data on vaccine preventable diseases and proposes recommendations for policies. No additional groups outside the government propose recommendations. Recommendations must be approved by the Commission of Public Health and then by the Inter-Territorial Council, at which point they are incorporated into the National Immunization Schedule.

The Spanish Association of Pediatrics, in conjunction with the Spanish Medicines Agency, outlines specifications for vaccination schedules and policies and provides a history of vaccination policies implemented in the past, as well as legislature pertaining to the public currently. Spain's Constitution does not mandate vaccination, so it is voluntary unless authorities require compulsory vaccination in the case of epidemics. In 1921 vaccination became mandatory for smallpox, and in 1944 the Bases Health Act mandated compulsory vaccination for diphtheria and smallpox, but was suspended in 1979 after the elimination of the threat of an epidemic. The first systematic immunization schedule for the provinces of Spain was established in 1975 and has continuously been updated by each autonomous community in regard to doses at certain ages and recommendation of additional vaccine not proposed in the schedule. The 2015 schedule proposed the newest change with the inclusion of pneumococcal vaccine for children under 12 months. For 2016, the schedule plans to propose a vaccine against varicella in children at 12–15 months and 3–4 years. Furthermore, the General Health Law of 1986 echoes Article 40.2 from the Constitution guaranteeing the right to the protection of health, and states employers must provide vaccines to workers if they are at risk of exposure. Due to vaccination coverage in each Community, there is little anti-vaccine activity or opposition to the current schedule, and no organized groups against vaccines. The universal public health care provides coverage for all residents, while central and regional support programs extend coverage to immigrant populations. However, no national funds are granted to the Communities for vaccine purchases. Vaccines are financed from taxes, and paid in full by the Community government. Law 21 in Article 2.6 establishes the need for proper clinical documentation and informed consent by the patient, although written informed consent is not mandated in the verbal request of a vaccine for a minor. The autonomous regions collect data, from either electronic registries or written physician charts, to calculate immunization coverage.

Tanzania

According to the World Health Organization vaccination coverage in Tanzania was more than 90% in 2012. An Electronic Immunisation Register has been established, which permits online access to the medical records of mothers and infants, enabling vaccination teams in remote areas to operate more effectively, especially with nomadic people. It also helps to coordinate stock levels and order new supplies.

United States

The Advisory Committee on Immunization Practices makes scientific recommendations which are generally followed by the federal government, state governments, and private health insurance companies.

All 50 states in the U.S. mandate immunizations for children in order to enroll in public school, but various exemptions are available depending on the state. All states have exemptions for people who have medical contraindications to vaccines, and all states except for California, West Virginia, and Mississippi allow religious exemptions, while eighteen states allow parents to cite personal, conscientious, philosophical, or other objections. An increasing number of parents are using religious and philosophical exemptions: researchers have cited this increased use of exemptions as contributing to loss of herd immunitywithin these communities, and hence an increasing number of disease outbreaks.

The American Academy of Pediatrics (AAP) advises physicians to respect the refusal of parents to vaccinate their child after adequate discussion, unless the child is put at significant risk of harm (e.g., during an epidemic, or after a deep and contaminated puncture wound). Under such circumstances, the AAP states that parental refusal of immunization constitutes a form of medical neglect and should be reported to state child protective services agencies.

Immunizations are often compulsory for military enlistment in the U.S.

All vaccines recommended by the U.S. government for its citizens are required for green card applicants. This requirement stirred controversy when it was applied to the HPV vaccine in July 2008 because of the cost of the vaccine, and because the other thirteen required vaccines prevent diseases which are spread by a respiratory route and are considered highly contagious, while HPV is only spread through sexual contact. In November 2009, this requirement was canceled.

Schools

The United States has a long history of school vaccination requirements. The first school vaccination requirement was enacted in the 1850s in Massachusetts to prevent the spread of smallpox. The school vaccination requirement was put in place after the compulsory school attendance law caused a rapid increase in the number of children in public schools, increasing the risk of smallpox outbreaks. The early movement towards school vaccination laws began at the local level including counties, cities, and boards of education. By 1827, Boston had become the first city to mandate that all children entering public schools show proof of vaccination. In addition, in 1855 the Commonwealth of Massachusetts had established its own statewide vaccination requirements for all students entering school, this influenced other states to implement similar statewide vaccination laws in schools as seen in New York in 1862, Connecticut in 1872, Pennsylvania in 1895, and later the Midwest, South and Western US. By 1963, 20 states had school vaccination laws.

These vaccination laws resulted in political debates throughout the United States. An example of this political controversy occurred in 1893 in Chicago, where less than 10 percent of the children were vaccinated despite the twelve year old state law. Resistance was seen at the local level of the school district as some local school boards and superintendents opposed the state vaccination laws, leading the state board health inspectors to examine vaccination policies in schools. Resistance proceeded during the mid-1900s and in 1977 a nationwide Childhood Immunization Initiative was developed with the goal of increasing vaccination rates among children to 90% by 1979. During the two-year period of observation, the initiative reviewed the immunization records of more than 28 million children and vaccinated children who had not received the recommended vaccines.

In 1922 the constitutionality of childhood vaccination was examined in the Supreme Court case Zucht v. King. The court decided that a school could deny admission to children who failed to provide a certification of vaccination for the protection of the public health. In 1987, a measles epidemic occurred in Maricopa County, Arizona and another court case, Maricopa County Health Department vs. Harmon, examined the arguments of an individual's right to education over the states need to protect against the spread of disease. The court decided that it is prudent to take action to combat the spread of disease by denying un-vaccinated children a place in school until the risk for the spread of measles had passed.

Schools in the United States require an updated immunization record for all incoming and returning students. While all states require an immunization record, this does not mean that all students must get vaccinated. Opt-out criteria is determined at a state level. In the United States, opt-outs take one of three forms: medical, in which a vaccine is contraindicated due to a component ingredient allergy or existing medical condition; religious; and personal philosophical opposition. As of 2015, 47 states allow religious exemptions, with some states requiring proof of religious membership. Only Mississippi, West Virginia and California do not permit religious exemptions. 18 states allow personal or philosophical opposition to vaccination.

Mandatory vaccinations have received criticism. Parents say that vaccine mandates prevent one's right to choose, especially if the vaccinations could be harmful. 18 states allow personal or philosophical opposition to vaccination. Many states have increased their immunization exemption laws to fit those who do not believe in immunization mandates.

War

Judge's cartoon of Rudyard Kipling's famous poem "The White Man's Burden" published in 1899. The poem's philosophy quickly was utilized to explain/justify the United States response to annexation of the Philippines. The United States used the "white man's burden" as an argument for imperial control of the Philippines and Puerto Rico on the basis of moral necessity to ensure the spread of civility and modernity.

The United States has a very complex history with compulsory vaccination, particularly in enforcing compulsory vaccinations both domestically and abroad to protect American soldiers during times of war. There are hundreds of thousands of examples of soldier deaths that were not the result of combat wounds, but were instead from disease. Among wars with high death tolls from disease is the Civil War where an estimated 620,000 soldiers died from disease. American soldiers in other countries have spread diseases that ultimately disrupted entire societies and healthcare systems with famine and poverty.

7

Ethics in Pharmaceutical Sales

The ethics involved within pharmaceutical sales is built from the organizational ethics, which is a matter of system compliance, accountability and culture (Grace & Cohen, 2005). Organizational ethics are used when developing the marketing and sales strategy to both the public and the healthcare profession of the strategy. Organizational ethics are best demonstrated through acts of fairness, compassion, integrity, honor, and responsibility.

Industry

The pharmaceutical industry is a highly competitive business and its success is dependent on the sales and marketing of each drug. The cost of research and development for each drug is hundreds of millions of dollars. In 2005 the research and development expenditure for the biopharmaceutical industry within Europe and the US was 15,474 million euro.(The Pharma Industry Figures, 2006). Some health economists peg the current cost of drug development at US$1.3 billion, others at US$1.7 billion The actual drug discovery and the drug development can take years. After which, testing and clinical trials are required prior to getting approval by regulatory boards. After launching the drug the company has much at stake as it has already outlaid millions of dollars the success of its sales is an important factor to the success of the company.

Sales Practices

A pharmaceutical sales representative is the key part within the sales of all drugs. They ensure the healthcare profession is informed of the benefits of the drug along with the safety and the side effects according to the dictate of the company employing them. The term used is ethical promotion, which can be described as communication of ethical values to promote their product to the physician. (Wright

& Lundstrom, 2004)

Regulations and Guidelines

European Federation of Pharmaceutical Industries and Associations

The European Federation of Pharmaceutical Industries and Associations (EFPIA) stipulates that there is a Corporate Social responsibility for the pharmaceutical industry to recognize and acknowledge the need to act responsibly towards society and the communities in which it operates.

The EFPIA has also code of practice on the promotion of medicine, which entails the regulations over many areas of the promotion of medicine. These include events and hospitality that can be extended by a pharmaceutical company. Gifts and inducements must be inexpensive and provide value to the practice of medicine or pharmacy. All medical sales representatives must have the adequate training and sufficient scientific knowledge to provide relevant and precise information about the products. They must also comply with the requirements of the applicable codes.

Pharmaceutical Research and Manufacturers of America

In 2002 the Pharmaceutical Research and Manufacturers of America, issued a set of guidelines for its member companies to follow when it comes to the relationship between drug reps and doctors. The voluntary code significantly changed how drug company representatives interact with doctors. Changes range from restricting gifts to limiting consulting contracts offered to doctors.

PhRMA was inspired to come up with the code after years of criticism from groups like Families USA and Public Citizen. PhRMA already had a set of guidelines on this topic but its board decided that one of the best ways to thwart the criticism and prevent any appearance of impropriety was to come up with a stricter code.

"The PhRMA guidelines are one major factor contributing to a paradigm shift that directly impacts the way our industry conducts business,""Because of this shift, pharmaceutical sales forces must learn new and more compelling ways to create and keep customers, or perish because physicians are no longer willing to listen to their usual approach," said Susan Torroella, CEO of Columbia MedCom Group.

PhRMA is opposed to state laws that regulate interaction between pharmaceutical sales representatives and health care providers. PhRMA officials said state regulations could create a patchwork of conflicting rules across the states that might do more to confuse sales representatives and doctors than prevent improper perks."We do have the comprehensive guidelines combined with the guidelines of the Office of Inspector General. Not only would state laws be a duplication, it could be nightmarish because you would have differing standards for different states," said Jeff Trewhitt, a spokesman for PhRMA.

U.S. Department of Health and Human Services

After PhRMA enacted its guidelines, the Office of Inspector General for the U.S. Department of Health and Human Services issued guidelines similar to PhRMA's code, except with more severe penalties. Companies that fail to follow the department's rules could face a federal investigation that could lead to civil penalties.

Health care Fraud

Pharmaceutical fraud involves activities that result in false claims to insurers or programs such as Medicare in the United States or equivalent state programs for financial gain to a pharmaceutical company. There are several different schemes used to defraud the health care system which are particular to the pharmaceutical industry. These include: Good Manufacturing Practice (GMP) Violations, Off Label Marketing, Best Price Fraud, CME Fraud, Medicaid Price Reporting, and Manufactured Compound Drugs. The Federal Bureau of Investigation (FBI) estimates that health care fraud costs American taxpayers $60 billion a year. Of this amount $2.5 billion was recovered through False Claims Act cases in FY 2010. Examples of fraud cases include the Pfizer $2.3 billion settlement and Merck $650 million settlement. Damages from fraud can be recovered by use of the False Claims Act, most commonly under the qui tam provisions which rewards an individual for being a "whistleblower", or relator (law).

Antipsychotic drugs are now the top-selling class of pharmaceuticals in America, generating annual revenue of about $14.6 billion. Every major company selling the drugs — Bristol-Myers Squibb, Eli Lilly, Pfizer, AstraZeneca and Johnson & Johnson — has either settled recent government cases, under the False Claims Act, for hundreds of millions of dollars or is currently under investigation for possible health care fraud. Following charges of illegal marketing, two of the settlements set records last year for the largest criminal fines ever imposed on corporations. One involved Eli Lilly's antipsychotic Zyprexa, and the other involved Bextra. In the Bextra case, the government also charged Pfizer with illegally marketing another antipsychotic, Geodon; Pfizer settled that part of the claim for $301 million, without admitting any wrongdoing.

On 2 July 2012, GlaxoSmithKline pleaded guilty to criminal charges and agreed to a $3 billion settlement of the largest health-care fraud case in the U.S. and the largest payment by a drug company. The settlement is related to the company's illegal promotion of prescription drugs, its failure to report safety data, bribing doctors, and promoting medicines for uses for which they were not licensed. The drugs involved were Paxil, Wellbutrin, Advair, Lamictal, and Zofran for off-label, non-covered uses. Those and the drugs Imitrex, Lotronex, Flovent, and Valtrex were involved in the kickback scheme.

United States Department of Health and Human Services

The United States Department of Health and Human Services (HHS), is a cabinet-level executive branch department of the U.S. federal government created to protect the health of all Americans and providing essential human services. Its motto is "Improving the health, safety, and well-being of America". Before the separate federal Department of Education was created in 1979, it was called the Department of Health, Education, and Welfare (HEW).

HHS is administered by the Secretary of Health and Human Services, who is appointed by the president with the advice and consent of the United States Senate. The position is currently held by Xavier Becerra.

The United States Public Health Service Commissioned Corps, the uniformed service of the PHS, is led by the Surgeon General who is responsible for addressing matters concerning public health as authorized by the secretary or by the Assistant Secretary of Health in addition to his or her primary mission of administering the Commissioned Corps.

Federal Security Agency

The Federal Security Agency (FSA) was established on July 1, 1939, under the Reorganization Act of 1939, P.L. 76–19. The objective was to bring together in one agency all federal programs in the fields of health, education, and social security. The first Federal Security Administrator was Paul V. McNutt. The new agency originally consisted of the following major components: (1) Office of the Administrator, (2) Public Health Service (PHS), (3) Office of Education, (4) Civilian Conservation Corps, and (5) Social Security Board.

By 1953, the Federal Security Agency's programs in health, education, and social security had grown to such importance that its annual budget exceeded the combined budgets of the Departments of Commerce, Justice, Labor, and Interior and affected the lives of millions of people. Consequently, in accordance with the Reorganization Act of 1949, President Eisenhower submitted to the Congress on March 12, 1953, Reorganization Plan No. 1 of 1953, which called for the dissolution of the Federal Security Agency and elevation of the agency to Cabinet status as the Department of Health, Education, and Welfare. The plan was approved on April 1, 1953, and became effective on April 11, 1953.

Unlike statutes authorizing the creation of other executive departments, the contents of Reorganization Plan No. 1 of 1953 were never properly codified within the United States Code, although Congress did codify a later statute ratifying the Plan. Today, the Plan is included as an appendix to Title 5 of the United States Code. The result is that HHS is the only executive department whose statutory foundation today rests on a confusing combination of several codified and uncodified statutes.

Department of Health, Education, and Welfare

The Department of Health, Education, and Welfare (HEW) was created on April 11, 1953, when Reorganization Plan No. 1 of 1953 became effective. HEW thus became the first new Cabinet-level department since the Department of Labor was created in 1913. The Reorganization Plan abolished the FSA and transferred all of its functions to the secretary of HEW and all components of the agency to the department. The first secretary of HEW was Oveta Culp Hobby, a native of Texas, who had served as commander of the Women's Army Corps in World War II and was editor and publisher of the Houston Post. Sworn in on April 11, 1953, as secretary, she had been FSA administrator since January 21, 1953.

The six major program-operating components of the new department were the Public Health Service, the Office of Education, the Food and Drug Administration, the Social Security Administration, the Office of Vocational Rehabilitation, and St. Elizabeth's Hospital. The department was also responsible for three federally aided corporations: Howard University, the American Printing House for the Blind, and the Columbia Institution for the Deaf (Gallaudet College since 1954).

Department of Health & Human Services

The Department of Health, Education, and Welfare was renamed the Department of Health & Human Services (HHS) in 1979, when its education functions were transferred to the newly created United States Department of Education under the Department of Education Organization Act. HHS was left in charge of the Social Security Administration, agencies constituting the Public Health Service, and Family Support Administration.

In 1995, the Social Security Administration was removed from the Department of Health & Human Services, and established as an independent agency of the executive branch of the United States Government.

The 2010 United States federal budget established a reserve fund of more than $630 billion over 10 years to finance fundamental reform of the health care system.

Organization

Internal structure

The Department of Health & Human Services is led by the United States Secretary of Health and Human Services, a member of the United States Cabinet appointed by the President of the United States with the consent of the United States Senate. The secretary is assisted in managing the department by the Deputy Secretary of Health and Human Services, who is also appointed by the president. The secretary and deputy secretary are further assisted by seven assistant secretaries, who serve as top departmental administrators.

As of January 20, 2018, this is the top level of the organizational chart. HHS provides further organizational detail on its website.

Several agencies within HHS are components of the U.S. Public Health Service (PHS), as noted below.

Immediate Office of the Secretary

The Immediate Office of the Secretary (IOS) is the top-level unit that directly reports to the Secretary of Health and Human Services. They assist in the administration of HHS and include the following components:

Office of the Deputy Secretary (DS) - an Executive Schedule, Level II Position. This role is responsible for all departmental operations.

Office of the Chief of Staff (COS) - This role is responsible for staff coordination and support.

Office of the General Counsel (OGC)

Executive Secretariat (ES or ExecSec) - Develops and reviews rules, regulations, correspondences, Reports to Congress, and other policy-related documents and decisions. Headed by the Executive Secretary to the Department and assisted by the Deputy Executive Secretary Deputy Executive Secretary.

Office of Health Reform - Oversees the implementation of new policies and legislation.

Office of the Chief Technology Officer (CTO) - Oversees the use of Data and Technology implementations in HHS.

Office of National Security (ONS) - A department-wide office that provides oversight, policy direction, standards, and performance assessments on all intelligence and national security related programs within HHS.

Office of the Secretary

The Office of the Secretary (OS) is the unit directly below the Immediate Office of the Secretary, but still directly reports to the Secretary. This unit consists of the offices of assistant secretaries including:

Office of the Assistant Secretary of Health and Human Services for Financial Resources (ASFR)

Office of the National Coordinator for Health Information Technology (ONC)

Office of the Assistant Secretary of Health and Human Services for Public Affairs (ASPA)

Office of the Assistant Secretary for Legislation (ASL)

Office of the Assistant Secretary of Health and Human Services for Planning and Evaluation (ASPE)

Office of Intergovernmental and External Affairs

The Office of Intergovernmental and External Affairs (IEA) serves as the liaison to state, local and tribal governments as well as NGOs. Through the IEA, HHS directs oversees current federal health programs at the regional and tribal level.

Headquarters Staff - assists the HHS Secretary in developing policies related to state and local government relations.

Tribal Affairs - serves as the point of contact for HHS regarding HHS programs on Indian reservations.

Center for Faith-based and Neighborhood Partnerships (a.k.a. the Partnership Center) - works to create partnerships with faith-based and community organizations at the local level.

Office of Human Resources - the department-wide office for HR related issues.

Office of Inspector General

\The Office of Inspector General, U.S. Department of Health and Human Services (OIG) investigates criminal activity for HHS. The special agents who work for OIG have the same title series "1811" as other federal criminal investigators, such as the FBI, HSI, ATF, DEA and Secret Service. They receive their law enforcement training at the U.S. Department of Homeland Security's Federal Law Enforcement Training Center in Glynco, Georgia. OIG Special Agents have special skills in investigating white collar crime related to Medicare and Medicaid fraud and abuse. Organized crime has dominated the criminal activity relative to this type of fraud.

HHS-OIG investigates tens of millions of dollars in Medicare fraud each year. In addition, OIG will continue its coverage of all 50 states and the District of Columbia by its multi-agency task forces (PSOC Task Forces) that identify, investigate, and prosecute individuals who willfully avoid payment of their child support obligations under the Child Support Recovery Act.

HHS-OIG agents also provide protective services to the Secretary of HHS, and other department executives as necessary.

In 2002, the department released Healthy People 2010, a national strategic initiative for improving the health of Americans.

With the passage of the Fraud Enforcement and Recovery Act of 2009, and the Affordable Care Act of 2010, the Office of the Inspector General has taken an emboldened stance against healthcare related non-compliance, most notably for violations of Stark Law and the Anti-Kickback Statute.

In 2015, the OIG issued a fraud alert as a warning to hospitals and healthcare systems to monitor and comply with their physician compensation arrangements.

Recent years have seen dramatic increases in both the number and the amounts of Stark Law violation settlements, prompting healthcare experts to identify a need for automated solutions that manage physician arrangements by centralizing necessary information with regard to physician–hospital integration. Contract management software companies such as Meditract provide options for health systems to organize and store physician contracts. Ludi Inc introduced DocTime Log®, an SaaS solution that specifically addresses this growing concern, automating physician time logging in compliance with contract terms to eliminate Stark Law and Anti-Kickback Statute violations.

According to a report released by the OIG in July 2019, more than 80 percent of the 4,563 U.S. hospice centers that provide care to Medicare beneficiaries surveyed from 2012 to 2016 have at least one deficiency and 20 percent have at least one "serious deficiency".

From January 2020, Christi Grimm became the principal deputy inspector general. She assumed the duties of an acting inspector general, because the inspector general post was empty. In April 2020, Grimm released a report which surveyed the state of hospitals in late March during the COVID-19 pandemic in the United States. The hospitals reported "severe shortages of testing supplies", "frequently waiting 7 days or longer for test results", which extended the length of patient stays and strained resources, and "widespread shortages of PPE". President Trump called the report "wrong" and questioned Grimm's motives. Later he called the report "Another Fake Dossier!" In May 2020, Trump nominated Jason Weida to be the permanent inspector general, pending confirmation by the U.S. Senate. According to a department spokeswoman, Grimm will remain as principal deputy inspector general.

Programs

The Department of Health & Human Services' administers 115 programs across its 11 operating divisions. The United States Department of Health & Human Services (HHS) aims to "protect the health of all Americans and provide essential human services, especially for those who are least able to help themselves." These federal programs consist of social service programs, civil rights and healthcare privacy programs, disaster preparedness programs, and health related research. HHS offers a variety of social service programs geared toward persons with low income, disabilities, military families, and senior citizens. Healthcare rights are defined under HHS in the Health Insurance Portability and Accountability Act (HIPAA) which protect patient's privacy in regards to medical information, protects workers health insurance when unemployed, and sets guidelines surrounding some health insurance. HHS collaborates with the Office of the Assistant Secretary for Preparedness and Response and Office of Emergency Management to prepare and respond to health emergencies. A broad array of health related research is supported or completed under the HHS; secondarily under HHS, the Health Resources & Service Administration houses data warehouses and makes health data available surrounding a multitude of topics. HHS also has vast offering of health related resources and tools to help educate the public on health policies and pertinent population health information. Some examples of available resources include disease prevention, wellness, health insurance information, as well as links to healthcare providers and facilities, meaningful health related materials, public health and safety information.

Some highlights include

Health and social science research

Preventing disease, including immunization services

Assuring food and drug safety

Medicare (health insurance for elderly and disabled Americans) and Medicaid (health insurance for low-income people)

Health information technology

Financial assistance and services for low-income families

Improving maternal and infant health, including a Nurse Home Visitation to support first-time mothers

Head Start (pre-school education and services)

Faith-based and community initiatives

Preventing child abuse and domestic violence

Substance abuse treatment and prevention

Services for older Americans, including home-delivered meals

Comprehensive health services for Native Americans

Assets for Independence

Medical preparedness for emergencies, including potential terrorism

Child support enforcement

The Health Insurance Portability and Accountability Act (HIPAA)

This program is to ensure the accountability of medical professionals to respect and carry-out basic human health rights, under the act of the same name. In the United States, the government feels that it is essential for the American people to understand their civil duty and rights to all of their medical information. That includes: health insurance policies or medical records from every doctor or emergency visit in one's life. Through Health & Human services one is able to file a complaint that their HIPAA rights have been violated or a consultant that will be able to decide if their rights were violated.

Social Services

This branch has everything to do with the social justice, wellness, and care of all people throughout the United States. This includes but is not limited to people who need government assistance, foster care, unaccompanied alien children, daycares (headstart included), adoption, senior citizens, and disability programs. Social services is one of (if not) the largest branch of programs underneath it that has a wide variety throughout the United States at a state and local level.

Prevention and Wellness

The prevention and wellness program's main idea is to give the American people the ability to live the healthiest and best lifestyle physically that they can. They are the ones who deal with vaccines and immunizations, which fight from common diseases to deadly ones. The nutrition & fitness program that are the basics of healthy eating and regular exercise. Health screenings & family health history which are crucial in the knowledge of each individual's health and body. A severely important one especially in today's society is mental health and substance abuse in where they help people with mental illness and drug abuse. Lastly, they help with environmental health where people are researching and studying how our environments both physical and metaphorically have a short- and long-term effect on our health and wellness.

Strengthening Communities Fund

In June 2010, the Department of Health & Human Services created the Strengthening Communities Fund as part of the American Recovery and Reinvestment Act. The fund was appropriated $50 million to be given as grants to organizations in the United States who were engaged in Capacity Building programs. The grants were given to two different types of capacity builders:

State, Local and Tribal governments engaged in capacity building: grants will go to state local and tribal governments to equip them with the capacity to more effectively partner with faith-based or non-faith based nonprofit organizations. Capacity building in this program will involve education and outreach that catalyzes more involvement of nonprofit organizations in economic recovery and building up nonprofit organization's abilities to tackle economic problems. State, Local and Tribal governments can receive up to $250,000 in two year grants

Nonprofit Social Service Providers engaged in capacity building: they will make grants available to nonprofit organizations who can assist other nonprofit organizations in organizational development, program development, leadership, and evaluations. Nonprofits can receive up to $1 million in two year grants

Biodefense

HHS plays a role in protecting the United States against bioterrorism events. In 2018, HHS released a new National Biodefense Strategy required by passage of the 2016 Biodefense Strategy Act. The Biodefense Strategy required implementation of a biodefense strategy after a 2015 Blue Ribbon Study Panel on Biodefense report found that the 2009 National Strategy for Countering Biological Threats was inadequate in protecting the U.S. The strategy adopted these five central recommendations: creating a single centralized approach to biodefense; implementing an interdisciplinary approach to biodefense that brings together policy makers, scientists, health experts, and academics; drawing up a comprehensive strategy to address human, plant, and animal health; creating a defense against global and domestic biological threats; and creating a proactive policy to combat the misuse and abuse of advanced biotechnology.

HHS also runs the Biodefense Steering Committee, which works with other federal agencies including the U.S. Department of State, U.S. Department of Defense, U.S. Food and Drug Administration, U.S. Department of Homeland Security, and the Environmental Protection Agency. HHS specifically oversees Project BioShield, established in 2003 and operating since 2004, and its development and production of genetically based bio-weapons and vaccines. HHS together with DHS are authorized under the Homeland Security Act of 2002 to deploy the weapons and vaccines produced by Project BioShield on the US general public under martial law during "emerging terrorist threats" or public health emergencies. Both HHS and DHS have similar authorities through state-based legislation adopted from Model State Emergency Health Powers Act provisions.

Criticisms and Controversies

In 2016, a published US Senate report revealed that several dozen unaccompanied children from Central America, some as young as 14 years old, were released from custody to traffickers where they were sexually assaulted, starved or forced to work for little or no pay. The HHS sub agency Office of Refugee Resettlement (ORR) released approximately 90,000 unaccompanied children during 2013–2015 but did not track their whereabouts or properly screen families accepting these children.

To prevent similar episodes, the Homeland Security and Health & Human Services Departments signed a memorandum of understanding in 2016, and agreed to establish joint procedures within one year for dealing with unaccompanied migrant children. As of 2018 they have failed to do so. Between October and December 2017, officials from ORR tried to contact 7,635 children and their sponsors. From these calls, officials learned that 6,075 children remained with their sponsors. Twenty-eight had run away, five had been removed from the United States and fifty-two had relocated to live with a non sponsor. However, officials have lost track of 1,475 children. ORR claims it is not legally liable for the safety and status of the childrenonce released from custody.

HHS is evidenced to be actively coercing and forcing bio-substances such as antipsychotics on migrating children without consent, and under questionable medical supervision. Medical professionals state that wrongly prescribed antipsychotics are especially dangerous for children, and can cause permanent psychological damage.

Medical professionals also state DHS and HHS incarceration and separation policies are likewise causing irreparable mental harm to the children.

Children are also dying in HHS custody. The forced drugging, deaths, and disappearances of migrating Mexican and Central American children might be related to DHS falsely labeling them and their families as 'terror threats' before HHS manages their incarcerations. Despite a federal court order, the DHS separation practices started by Obama and mandated by the Trump administration's "zero-tolerance" policy have not been halted, and HHS has not stopped forcing drugs on the children it incarcerates.

Freedom of Information Act Processing Performance

In the latest Center for Effective Government analysis of 15 federal agencies which receive the most Freedom of Information Act (FOIA) requests published in 2015 (using 2012 and 2013 data, the most recent years available), the DHHS ranked second to last, earning an F by scoring 57 out of a possible 100 points, largely due to a low score on its particular disclosure rules. It had deteriorated from a D- in 2013.

Pharmaceutical sales representative

Pharmaceutical sales representatives (formerly detailmen) are salespeople employed by pharmaceutical companies to persuade doctors to prescribe their drugs to patients. Drug companies in the United States spend ~$5 billion annually sending representatives to doctors, to provide product information, answer questions on product use, and deliver product samples. These interactions are governed according to limits established by the Code on Interactions with Health Care Professionals, created by the Pharmaceutical Research and Manufacturers of America (PhRMA). This code came into practice in 2002 and has since been updated to help define ethical interactions between health care professionals and the pharmaceutical companies

Companies maintain this provides an educational service by keeping doctors updated on the latest changes in medical science. Critics point to a systematic use of gifts and personal information to befriend doctors to influence their drug prescriptions. In the United Kingdom representatives are governed by a strict code of conduct from the Association of British Pharmaceutical Industries (ABPI). No gifts are allowed. Companies are fined and held in breach if they use the tactics described in this description.

Methods

Doctors can receive small gifts, such as free dinners, event or travel tickets, clocks, free drug samples and swag. Controversial inducements include jobs offers for the drug company, consulting / speaking fees, and all-expense-paid travel to resorts and exotic locations where attendance is limited or not mandatory.

Pharmaceutical Representative is a trade journal featuring common sales tactics such as how to close a tough sale by flattering a stubborn doctor. Along with flattery, the attractiveness of sales reps has been noted, with a trend of former cheerleaders entering the field. Researchers note; "seduction appeared to be a deliberate industry strategy", and in informal survey by a doctor found that 12 out of 13 women sales reps said they had been sexually harassed by doctors.

Me-too Drugs

Sales reps push new "follow on" or "me-too" drugs with free samples that are more expensive than existing generic drugs, such as Nexium which costs three times as much as its predecessor Prilosec, with no evidence of improved efficacy. With beta-blockers and statins, me-too drugs have improved results, and increased competition while lowering prices. As me-too drugs are similar but new, their side effects can be unknown and not well understood. Pharmaceutical marketing / reps assert a me-too drug may work better than another, but they "don't test their me-too drugs in people who have not done well with an earlier drug of the same class."

Laws

In 1990, the Food and Drug Administration (FDA) passed laws banning "gifts of substantial value" of drug companies to doctors, however this has changed the gifts from objects to meals and travel.

In 2006, New Hampshire forbid the sale of prescription data to commercial entities.

Encountering ill-informed reps at his practice Dr. Dan Foster, a West Virginia surgeon and lawmaker, introduced a bill to require reps to have science degrees. While it did not pass, it led to a disclosure of minimum hiring requirements.

Alternatives

In Australia the government funds academic detailers that are impartial medical students who provide drug information to medical professionals.

Culture

Cheerleading athletes have been noted as a recruitment target by companies to hire as pharmaceutical sales representatives.

8

Drug Development

Drug development is the process of bringing a new pharmaceutical drug to the market once a lead compound has been identified through the process of drug discovery. It includes preclinical research on microorganisms and animals, filing for regulatory status, such as via the United States Food and Drug Administration for an investigational new drug to initiate clinical trials on humans, and may include the step of obtaining regulatory approval with a new drug application to market the drug. The entire process – from concept through preclinical testing in the laboratory to clinical trial development, including Phase I–III trials – to approved vaccine or drug typically takes more than a decade.

New Chemical Entity Evelopment

Broadly, the process of drug development can be divided into preclinical and clinical work.

Pre-Clinical

New chemical entities (NCEs, also known as new molecular entities or NMEs) are compounds that emerge from the process of drug discovery. These have promising activity against a particular biological target that is important in disease. However, little is known about the safety, toxicity, pharmacokinetics, and metabolism of this NCE in humans. It is the function of drug development to assess all of these parameters prior to human clinical trials. A further major objective of drug development is to recommend the dose and schedule for the first use in a human clinical trial ("first-in-human" [FIH] or First Human Dose [FHD], previously also known as "first-in-man" [FIM]).

In addition, drug development must establish the physicochemical properties of the NCE: its chemical makeup, stability, and solubility. Manufacturers must optimize the process they use to make the chemical so they can scale up from a medicinal chemist producing milligrams, to manufacturing on the kilogram and ton scale. They further examine the product for suitability to package as capsules, tablets, aerosol, intramuscular injectable, subcutaneous injectable, or intravenous formulations. Together, these processes are known in preclinical and clinical development as chemistry, manufacturing, and control (CMC).

Many aspects of drug development focus on satisfying the regulatory requirements for a new drug application. These generally constitute a number of tests designed to determine the major toxicities of a novel compound prior to first use in humans. It is a legal requirement that an assessment of major organ toxicity be performed (effects on the heart and lungs, brain, kidney, liver and digestive system), as well as effects on other parts of the body that might be affected by the drug (e.g., the skin if the new drug is to be delivered on or through the skin). Such preliminary tests are made using in vitro methods (e.g., with isolated cells), but many tests can only use experimental animals to demonstrate the complex interplay of metabolism and drug exposure on toxicity.

The information is gathered from this preclinical testing, as well as information on CMC, and submitted to regulatory authorities (in the US, to the FDA), as an Investigational New Drug (IND) application. If the IND is approved, development moves to the clinical phase.

Clinical Phase

Clinical trials involve three or four steps:

Phase I trials, usually in healthy volunteers, determine safety and dosing.

Phase II trials are used to get an initial reading of efficacy and further explore safety in small numbers of patients having the disease targeted by the NCE.

Phase III trials are large, pivotal trials to determine safety and efficacy in sufficiently large numbers of patients with the targeted disease. If safety and efficacy are adequately proved, clinical testing may stop at this step and the NCE advances to the new drug application (NDA) stage.

Phase IV trials are post-approval trials that are sometimes a condition attached by the FDA, also called post-market surveillance studies.

The process of defining characteristics of the drug does not stop once an NCE is advanced into human clinical trials. In addition to the tests required to move a novel vaccine or antiviral drug into the clinic for the first time, manufacturers must ensure that any long-term or chronic toxicities are well-defined, including effects on systems not previously monitored (fertility, reproduction, immune system, among others).

If a vaccine candidate or antiviral compound emerges from these tests with an acceptable toxicity and safety profile, and the manufacturer can further show it has the desired effect in clinical trials, then the NCE portfolio of evidence can be submitted for marketing approval in the various countries where the manufacturer plans to sell it. In the United States, this process is called a "new drug application" or NDA.

Most novel drug candidates (NCEs) fail during drug development, either because they have unacceptable toxicity or because they simply do not prove efficacy on the targeted disease, as shown in Phase II–III clinical trials. Critical reviews of drug development programs indicate that Phase II–III clinical trials fail due mainly to unknown toxic side effects (50% failure of Phase II cardiology trials), and because of inadequate financing, trial design weaknesses, or poor trial execution.

A study covering clinical research in the 1980–90s found that only 21.5% of drug candidates that started Phase I trials were eventually approved for marketing. During 2006–15, the success rate of obtaining approval from Phase I to successful Phase III trials was under 10% on average, and 16% specifically for vaccines. The high failure rates associated with pharmaceutical development are referred to as an "attrition rate", requiring decisions during the early stages of drug development to "kill" projects early to avoid costly failures.

Cost

One 2010 study assessed both capitalized and out-of-pocket costs for bringing a single new drug to market as about US$1.8 billion and $870 million, respectively. A median cost estimate of 2015–16 trials for development of 10 anti-cancer drugs was $648 million. In 2017, the median cost of a pivotal trial across all clinical indications was $19 million.

The average cost (2013 dollars) of each stage of clinical research was US$25 million for a Phase I safety study, $59 million for a Phase II randomized controlled efficacy study, and $255 million for a pivotal Phase III trial to demonstrate its equivalence or superiority to an existing approved drug, possibly as high as $345 million. The average cost of conducting a 2015–16 pivotal Phase III trial on an infectious disease drug candidate was $22 million.

The full cost of bringing a new drug (i.e., new chemical entity) to market – from discovery through clinical trials to approval – is complex and controversial. In a 2016 review of 106 drug candidates assessed through clinical trials, the total capital expenditure for a manufacturer having a drug approved through successful Phase III trials was $2.6 billion (in 2013 dollars), an amount increasing at an annual rate of 8.5%. Over 2003–2013 for companies that approved 8–13 drugs, the cost per drug could rise to as high as $5.5 billion, due mainly to international geographic expansion for marketing and ongoing costs for Phase IV trials for continuous safety surveillance.

Alternatives to conventional drug development have the objective for universities, governments, and the pharmaceutical industry to collaborate and optimize resources. An example of a collaborative drug development initiative is COVID

Moonshot, an international open-science project started in March 2020 with the goal of developing an un-patented oral antiviral drug to treat SARS-CoV-2.

Valuation

The nature of a drug development project is characterised by high attrition rates, large capital expenditures, and long timelines. This makes the valuation of such projects and companies a challenging task. Not all valuation methods can cope with these particularities. The most commonly used valuation methods are risk-adjusted net present value (rNPV), decision trees, real options, or comparables.

The most important value drivers are the cost of capital or discount rate that is used, phase attributes such as duration, success rates, and costs, and the forecasted sales, including cost of goods and marketing and sales expenses. Less objective aspects like quality of the management or novelty of the technology should be reflected in the cash flows estimation.

Success Rate

Candidates for a new drug to treat a disease might, theoretically, include from 5,000 to 10,000 chemical compounds. On average about 250 of these show sufficient promise for further evaluation using laboratory tests, mice and other test animals. Typically, about ten of these qualify for tests on humans. A study conducted by the Tufts Center for the Study of Drug Development covering the 1980s and 1990s found that only 21.5 percent of drugs that started Phase I trials were eventually approved for marketing. In the time period of 2006 to 2015, the success rate was 9.6%. The high failure rates associated with pharmaceutical development are referred to as the "attrition rate" problem. Careful decision making during drug development is essential to avoid costly failures. In many cases, intelligent programme and clinical trial design can prevent false negative results. Well-designed, dose-finding studies and comparisons against both a placebo and a gold-standard treatment arm play a major role in achieving reliable data.

Computing Initiatives

Novel initiatives include partnering between governmental organizations and industry, such as the European Innovative Medicines Initiative. The US Food and Drug Administration created the "Critical Path Initiative" to enhance innovation of drug development, and the Breakthrough Therapy designation to expedite development and regulatory review of candidate drugs for which preliminary clinical evidence shows the drug candidate may substantially improve therapy for a serious disorder.

In March 2020, the United States Department of Energy, National Science Foundation, NASA, industry, and nine universities pooled resources to access supercomputers from IBM, combined with cloud computing resources from Hewlett Packard Enterprise, Amazon, Microsoft, and Google, for drug discovery. The

COVID-19 High Performance Computing Consortium also aims to forecast disease spread, model possible vaccines, and screen thousands of chemical compounds to design a COVID-19 vaccine or therapy. In May 2020, the OpenPandemics – COVID-19 partnership between Scripps Research and IBM's World Community Grid was launched. The partnership is a distributed computing project that "will automatically run a simulated experiment in the background [of connected home PCs] which will help predict the effectiveness of a particular chemical compound as a possible treatment for COVID-19".

Cost of drug development

The cost of drug development is the full cost of bringing a new drug (i.e., new chemical entity) to market from drug discovery through clinical trials to approval. Typically, companies spend tens to hundreds of millions of U.S. dollars on drug development. One element of the complexity is that the much-publicized final numbers often not only include the out-of-pocket expenses for conducting a series of Phase I-III clinical trials, but also the capital costs of the long period (10 or more years) during which the company must cover out-of-pocket costs for preclinical drug discovery. Additionally, companies often do not report whether a given figure includes the capitalized cost or comprises only out-of-pocket expenses, or both.

One study assessed both capitalized and out-of-pocket costs as about US$1.8 billion and $870 million, respectively.

In an analysis of the drug development costs for 98 companies over a decade, the average cost per drug developed and approved by a single-drug company was $350 million. But for companies that approved between eight and 13 drugs over 10 years, the cost per drug went as high as $5.5 billion, due mainly to geographic expansion for marketing and ongoing costs for Phase IV trials and continuous monitoring for safety.

A new study in 2020 estimated that the median cost of getting a new drug into the market was $985 million, and the average cost was $1.3 billion, which was much lower compared to previous studies, which have placed the average cost of drug development as $2.8 billion.

Alternatives to conventional drug development have the objective for universities, governments and pharmaceutical industry to collaborate and optimize resources.

Severin Schwan, the CEO of the Swiss company Roche, reported that Roche's research and development costs amounted to $12.3 billion in 2018, a quarter of the entire National Institutes of Health budget. Given the profit-driven nature of pharmaceutical companies and their research and development expenses, companies use their research and development expenses as a starting point to determine appropriate yet profitable prices.

Pharmaceutical companies spend a large amount on research and development before a drug is released to the market and costs can be further divided into three major fields: the discovery into the drug's specific medical field, clinical trials, and failed drugs.

Discovery

Drug discovery is the area of research and development that amounts to the most amount of time and money.[according to whom?] The process can involve scientists to determine the germs, viruses, and bacteria that cause a specific disease or illness. The time frame can range from 3–20 years and costs can range between several billion to tens of billions of dollars. Research teams attempt to break down disease components to find abnormal events/processes taking place in the body. Only then do scientists work on developing chemical compounds to treat these abnormalities with the aid of computer models.

After "discovery" and a creation of a chemical compound, pharmaceutical companies move forward with the Investigational New Drug (IND) Application from the FDA. After the investigation into the drug and given approval, pharmaceutical companies can move into pre-clinical trials and clinical trials.

Trials

Drug development and pre-clinical trials focus on non-human subjects and work on animals such as rats. This is the most inexpensive phase of testing.

The Food and Drug Administration mandates a 3 phase clinical trial testing that tests for side effects and the effectiveness of the drug with a single phase clinical trial costing upwards of $100 million.

After a drug has passed through all three phases, the pharmaceutical company can move forward with a New Drug Application from the FDA. In 2014, the FDA charged between $1 million to $2 million for an NDA.

Failed Drugs

The processes of "discovery" and clinical trials amounts to approximately 12 years from research lab to the patient, in which about 10% of all drugs that start pre-clinical trials ever make it to actual human testing. Each pharmaceutical company (which have hundreds of drugs moving in and out of these phases) will never recuperate the costs of "failed drugs". Thus, profits made from one drug need to cover the costs of previous "failed drugs".

Relationship

Overall, research and development expenses relating to a pharmaceutical drug amount to the billions. For example, it was reported that AstraZeneca spent upwards on average of $11 billion per drug for research and developmental purposes. The average of $11 billion only comprises the "discovery" costs, pre-clinical and clinical trial costs, and other expenses. With the addition of "failed drug" costs, the $11 billion easily amounts to over $20 billion in expenses. Therefore, an appropriate figure like $60 billion would be approximate sales figure that a pharmaceutical company like AstraZeneca would aim to generate to cover these costs and make a profit at the same time.

Total research and development costs provide pharmaceutical companies a ballpark estimation of total expenses. This is important in setting projected profit goals for a particular drug and thus, is one of the most necessary steps pharmaceutical companies take in pricing a particular drug.

Research on costs

Tufts Center for the Study of Drug Development has published numerous studies estimating the cost of developing new pharmaceutical drugs. In 2001, researchers from the Center estimated that the cost of doing so was $802 million, and in 2014, they released a study estimating that this amount had risen to nearly $2.6 billion. The 2014 study was criticized by Medecins Sans Frontieres, which said it was unreliable because the industry's research and development spending is not made public. Aaron Carroll of the New York Times also criticized the study, saying it "contains a lot of assumptions that tend to favor the pharmaceutical industry."

Orphan Drug

An orphan drug is a pharmaceutical agent developed to treat medical conditions which, because they are so rare, would not be profitable to produce without government assistance. The conditions are referred to as orphan diseases.

The assignment of orphan status to a disease and to drugs developed to treat it is a matter of public policy in many countries and has yielded medical breakthroughs that might not otherwise have been achieved, due to the economics of drug research and development.

In the U.S. and the EU, it is easier to gain marketing approval for an orphan drug. There may be other financial incentives, such as an extended period of exclusivity, during which the producer has sole rights to market the drug. All are intended to encourage development of drugs which would otherwise lack sufficient profit motive to attract corporate research budgets and personnel.

Definition

According to the US Food and Drug Administration (FDA), an orphan drug is defined as one "intended for the treatment, prevention or diagnosis of a rare disease or condition, which is one that affects less than 200,000 persons in the US" (which equates to approximately 6 cases per 10,000 population) "or meets cost recovery provisions of the act." In the European Union (EU), the European Medicines Agency (EMA) defines a drug as "orphan" if it is intended for the diagnosis, prevention or treatment of a life-threatening or chronically and seriously debilitating condition affecting not more than 5 in 10,000 EU people. EMA also qualifies a drug as orphan if – without incentives – it would be unlikely that marketing the drug in the EU would generate sufficient benefit for the affected people and for the drug manufacturer to justify the investment. As of 2017, there was no official integration of the orphan drug programs between the FDA and EMA.

Global Statistics

As of 2014, there were 281 marketed orphan drugs and more than 400 orphan designated drugs in clinical trials. More than 60% of orphan drugs were biologics. The U.S. dominated development of orphan drugs, with more than 300 in clinical trials, followed by Europe. Cancer treatment was the indication in more than 30% of orphan drug trials.

Number of orphan drugs in clinical trials: 600

Number of orphan drugs in phase 2 trial: 231

Number of orphan drugs in U.S. clinical trials: 350 in the pipeline from research until registration

Effect on Investment, Sales and Profit

According to Thomson Reuters in their 2012 publication "The Economic Power of Orphan Drugs", there has been increased investment in orphan drug research and development, partly due to the U.S. Orphan Drug Act of 1983 (ODA) and similar acts in other regions of the world driven by "high-profile philanthropic funding".

According to Drug Discovery Today, the years 2001 to 2011 were the "most productive period in the history of orphan drug development, in terms of average annual orphan drug designations and orphan drug approvals". :?660? For the same decade the compound annual growth rate (CAGR) of the orphan drugs was an "impressive 25.8%, compared to only 20.1% for a matched control group of non-orphan drugs". :?6? By 2012, the market for orphan drugs was worth US$637 million, compared with US$638 million for a control group of non-orphan drugs.

By 2012,

the revenue-generating potential of orphan drugs [was] as great as for non-orphan drugs, even though patient populations for rare diseases are significantly smaller. Moreover, we suggest that orphan drugs have greater profitability when considered in the full context of developmental drivers, including government financial incentives, smaller clinical trial sizes, shorter clinical trial times and higher rates of regulatory success.

—?Gaze and Breen 2012

According to a 2014 report, the orphan drug market has become increasingly lucrative for a number of reasons. The cost of clinical trials for orphan drugs is substantially lower than for other diseases because trial sizes are naturally much smaller than for more diseases with larger numbers of patients. Small clinical trials and minimal competition place orphan agents at an advantage in regulatory review.

Tax incentives reduce the cost of development. On average the cost per patient for orphan drugs is "six times that of non-orphan drugs, a clear indication of their pricing power". The cost of per-person outlays are large and are expected to increase with wider use of public subsidies.

The 2014 Orphan Drug report stated that the percentage of orphan drug sales as part of all prescription drug sales had been increasing at a rapid rate. The report projected a total of US$176 billion by 2020. Although orphan disease populations are the smallest, the cost of per-patient outlays among them are the largest and are expected to increase as more people with rare diseases become eligible for subsidies – in the U.S., for example, through the Affordable Care Act.

Legislation

Orphan drugs generally follow the same regulatory development path as any other pharmaceutical product, in which testing focuses on pharmacokinetics and pharmacodynamics, dosing, stability, safety and efficacy. However, some statistical burdens are lessened to maintain development momentum. For example, orphan drug regulations generally acknowledge the fact that it may not be possible to test 1,000 patients in a phase III clinical trial if fewer than that number are affected by the disease.

Government intervention on behalf of orphan drug development takes several forms:

Tax incentives

Exclusivity (enhanced patent protection and marketing rights)

Research subsidies

Creating a government-run enterprise to engage in research and development as in a Crown corporation

A 2015 study of "34 key Canadian stakeholders, including drug regulators, funders, scientists, policy experts, pharmaceutical industry representatives, and patient advocates" investigated factors behind the pharmaceutical industry growing interest in "niche markets" such as orphan drugs.

United States

The Orphan Drug Act (ODA) of January 1983, passed in the United States, with lobbying from the National Organization for Rare Disorders and many other organizations, is meant to encourage pharmaceutical companies to develop drugs for diseases that have a small market. Under the ODA drugs, vaccines, and diagnostic agents would qualify for orphan status if they were intended to treat a disease affecting fewer than 200,000 American citizens. Under the ODA orphan drug sponsors qualify for seven-year FDA-administered market Orphan Drug Exclusivity (ODE), "tax credits of up to 50% of R&D costs, R&D grants, waived FDA fees, protocol assistance :?660? and may get clinical trial tax incentives.

In the U.S., orphan drug designation means that the sponsor qualifies for certain benefits, but it does not mean the drug is safe, effective or legal.

In 2002, the Rare Diseases Act was signed into law. It amended the Public Health Service Act to establish the Office of Rare Diseases. It also increased funding for the development of treatments for people with rare diseases.

European Union

In 2000, the European Union (EU) enacted similar legislation, Regulation(EC) No 141/2000, which refers to drugs developed to treat rare diseases to as "orphan medicinal products". The EU's definition of an orphan condition is broader than that of the US, in that it also covers some tropical diseases that are primarily found in developing nations. Orphan drug status granted by the European Commission gives marketing exclusivity in the EU for 10 years after approval. The EU's legislation is administered by the Committee on Orphan Medicinal Products of the European Medicines Agency (EMA).

In late 2007 the FDA and EMA agreed to use a common application process for both agencies to make it easier for manufacturers to apply for orphan drug status but, while continuing two separate approval processes.

Other countries

Legislation has been implemented by Japan, Singapore, and Australia that offers subsidies and other incentives to encourage the development of drugs that treat orphan diseases.

Numbers of New Drugs

Under the ODA and EU legislation, many orphan drugs have been developed, including drugs to treat glioma, multiple myeloma, cystic fibrosis, phenylketonuria, snake venom poisoning, and idiopathic thrombocytopenic purpura.

The Pharmaceutical Executive opines, that the "ODA is nearly universally acknowledged to be a success".

Before the US Congress enacted the ODA in 1983, only 38 drugs were approved in the US specifically to treat orphan diseases. In the US, from January 1983 to June 2004, 249 orphan drugs received marketing authorization and 1,129 received different orphan drug designations, compared to fewer than ten such products in the decade prior to 1983. From 1983 until May 2010, the FDA approved 353 orphan drugs and granted orphan designations to 2,116 compounds. As of 2010, 200 of the roughly 7,000 officially designated orphan diseases have become treatable.

Critics have questioned whether orphan drug legislation was the real cause of this increase, claiming that many of the new drugs were for disorders which were already being researched anyway, and would have had drugs developed regardless of the legislation, and whether the ODA has truly stimulated the production of non-profitable drugs; the act also has been criticised for allowing some pharmaceutical companies to make a large profit off drugs which have a small market but sell for a high price.

While the European Medicines Agency grants orphan drugs market access in all member states, in practice, they only reach the market when a member state decides that its national health system will reimburse for the drug. For example, in 2008, 44 orphan drugs reached the market in the Netherlands, 35 in Belgium, and 28 in Sweden, while in 2007, 35 such drugs reached the market in France and 23 in Italy.

Though not technically an orphan disease, research and development into the treatment for AIDS has been heavily linked to the Orphan Drug Act. In the beginning of the AIDS epidemic the lack of treatment for the disease was often accredited to a believed lack of commercial base for a medication linked to HIV infection. This encouraged the FDA to use the Orphan Drug Act to help bolster research in this field, and by 1995 13 of the 19 drugs approved by the FDA to treat AIDS had received orphan drug designation, with 10 receiving marketing rights. These are in addition to the 70 designated orphan drugs designed to treat other HIV related illnesses.

Examples for Selected Diseases

Cystic fibrosis

In the 1980s, people with cystic fibrosis rarely lived beyond their early teens. Drugs like Pulmozyme and tobramycin, both developed with aid from the ODA, revolutionized treatment for cystic fibrosis patients by significantly improving their quality of life and extending their life expectancies. Now, cystic fibrosis patients often survive into their thirties and some into their fifties.

Familial Hypercholesterolemia

The 1985 Nobel Prize for medicine went to two researchers for their work related to fa4milial hypercholesterolemia, which causes large and rapid increases in cholesterol levels. Their research led to the development of statin drugs which are now commonly used to treat high cholesterol.

Wilson's Disease

Penicillamine was developed to treat Wilson's disease, a rare hereditary disease that can lead to a fatal accumulation of copper in the body. This drug was later found to be effective in treating arthritis. Bis-choline tetrathiomolybdate is currently under investigation as a therapy against Wilson's disease.

Phospholipase 2G6-Associated Neurodegeneration

In 2017, FDA granted RT001 orphan drug designation in the treatment of phospholipase 2G6-associated neurodegeneration (PLAN).

Transthyretin-Related Hereditary Amyloidosis

The FDA granted Patisiran (Onpattro) orphan drug status and breakthrough therapy designation due to its novel mechanism involving RNA therapy to block the production of an abnormal form of transthyretin. Patisiran received full FDA approval in 2018 and its RNA lipid nanoparticle drug delivery system was later used in the Pfizer–BioNTech COVID-19 vaccine and Moderna RNA vaccines.

Activism, Research Centers

The Center for Orphan Drug Research at the University of Minnesota College of Pharmacy helps small companies with insufficient in-house expertise and resources in drug synthesis, formulation, pharmacometrics, and bio-analysis. The Keck Graduate Institute Center for Rare Disease Therapies (CRDT) in Claremont, California, supports projects to revive potential orphan drugs whose development has stalled by identifying barriers to commercialization, such as problems with formulation and bio-processing.

Numerous advocacy groups such as the National Organization for Rare Disorders, Global Genes Project, Children's Rare Disease Network, Abetalipoproteinemia Collaboration Foundation, Zellweger Baby Support Network, and the Friedreich's Ataxia Research Alliance have been founded in order to advocate on behalf of patients with rare diseases with a particular emphasis on diseases that affect children.

Cost

According to a 2015 report published by EvaluatePharma, the economics of orphan drugs mirrors the economics of the pharmaceutical market as a whole but has a few very large differences. The market for orphan drugs is by definition very small, but while the customer base is drastically smaller the cost of research and development is very much the same as for non orphan drugs. This, the producers have claimed, causes them to charge extremely high amounts for treatment, sometimes as high as $700,000 a year, as in the case of Spinraza (Biogen), FDA approved in December 2016 for spinal muscular atrophy, placing a large amount of stress on insurance companies and patients. An analysis of 12 orphan drugs that were approved in the US between 1990 and 2000 estimated a price reduction of on average 50% upon loss of marketing exclusivity, with a range of price reductions from 14% to 95%.

Governments have implemented steps to reduce high research and development7cost with subsidies and other forms of financial assistance. The largest assistance are tax breaks which can be as high as 50% of research and development costs. Orphan drug manufacturers are also able to take advantage of the small customer base to cut cost on clinical trials due to the small number of cases to have smaller trials which reduces cost. These smaller clinical trials also allow orphan drugs to move to market faster as the average time to receive FDA approval for an orphan drug is 10 months compared to 13 months for non-orphan drugs. This is especially true in the market for cancer drugs, as a 2011 study found that between 2004 and 2010 orphan drug trials were more likely to be smaller and less randomized than their non-orphan counterparts, but still had a higher FDA approval rate, with 15 orphan cancer drugs being approved, while only 12 non-orphan drugs were approved. This allows manufactures to get cost to the point that it is economically feasible to produce these treatments. The subsidies can total up to $30 million per fiscal year in the United States alone.

By 2015, industry analysts and academic researchers agreed, that the sky-high price of orphan drugs, such as eculizumab, was not related to research, development and manufacturing costs. Their price is arbitrary and they have become more profitable than traditional medicines.

\Public resources went into understanding the molecular basis of the disease, public resources went into the technology to make antibodies and finally, Alexion, to their credit, kind of picked up the pieces.

—Sachdev Sidhu 2015

Public Funding

Evaluation criteria

By 2007 the use of economic evaluation methods regarding public-funding of orphan drugs, using estimates of the incremental cost-effectiveness, for example, became more established internationally. The QALY has often been used in cost-utility analysis to calculate the ratio of cost to QALYs saved for a particular health care intervention. By 2008 the National Institute for Health and Care Excellence (NICE) in England and Wales, for example, operated with a threshold range of £20,000–30,000 per quality-adjusted life year (QALY). By 2005 doubts were raised about the use of economic evaluations in orphan drugs. By 2008 most of the orphan drugs appraised had cost-effectiveness thresholds "well in excess of the 'accepted' level and would not be reimbursed according to conventional criteria". As early as 2005 McCabe et al. argued that rarity should not have a premium and orphan drugs should be treated like other pharmaceuticals in general. Drummond et al. argued that the social value of health technologies should also be included in the assessment along with the estimation of the incremental cost-effectiveness ratio.

Abuse Potential

The very large incentives given to pharmaceutical companies to produce orphan drugs have led to the impression that the financial support afforded to make these drugs possible is akin to abuse. Because drugs can be used to treat multiple conditions, companies can take drugs that were filed with their government agency as orphan drugs to receive financial assistance, and then market it to a wide population to increase their profit margin. For example AstraZeneca's cholesterol drug Crestor was filed as a treatment for the rare disease pediatric familial hypercholesterolemia. After the drug was approved for orphan drug designation, and AstraZeneca had received tax breaks and other advantages, AstraZeneca later applied and received FDA approval for the drug to be used to treat cholesterol in all diabetics.

NICE

The UK's National Institute for Health and Care Excellence (NICE) can pay from £100,000 to £300,000 per QALY (Quality Adjusted Life Year) for treatments of "very rare conditions". This is compared to under £20,000 for non-orphan drugs.

In 2015, NICE held consultations with "patient groups, the Department of Health, companies, learned societies, charities and researchers" regarding the appraisal of medicines and other technologies. There was a call for more research into new processes, including:

the model of pharmaceutical research and development, the expectations that companies and patient groups have about how risk and reward is shared between the industry and a publicly funded NHS, and in the arrangements for commissioning expensive new treatments.

— NICE 2014

9

Pharmaceutical Product Placement

Product placement is a well-established marketing technique that nevertheless continues to provoke considerable criticism and debate. Likewise, direct-to-patient marketing of pharmaceuticals is legally acceptable but is controversial among ethicists and medical professionals. Little has been published regarding the ethical challenges and pitfalls involved in medical marketing, including the issues of whether medical products should be treated differently from consumer products and whether pharmaceuticals are distinct from medical devices. Discussed are examples of pharmaceutical marketing as well as an episode from the Chicago Hope television program in which a medical device was touted as a solution for a problem for which the Food and Drug Administration (FDA) has not approved the use of the device. Legal and ethical considerations for product placement of medical products as they influence patient demand are also analyzed, as well as some of the pitfalls that may accompany direct marketing of medical products.

A POWERFUL MARKETING TOOL

Product placement advertising (also called stealth or subliminal advertising) is the insertion of a product or service into a script or scene of a TV show or movie, usually for a price negotiated with the network, producer, or scriptwriter. It has proven to be a highly effective method of marketing for a host of different products, from food to computers to cars. The overall market for product placement rose 3.5 percent to $3 billion in 2004, according to the paper's authors, professor Dominick Frosch and research assistant Sony Ta.

While controversy exists over how effective and ethical product placement is, most agree that as a marketing tool it has two big things going for it—it is relatively inexpensive, and is as-yet unregulated.

Pharmaceutical companies seem to have been slow to adopt product placement as part of their marketing mix. No pharma company has admitted having anything to do with the surge of drug mentions on TV shows. And only one company, Organon Pharmaceuticals, has openly embraced product placement. (To promote their NuvaRing contraceptive, they paid to have a poster appear in the examining room on the sitcom Scrubs.)

Why the reluctance? Frosch believes it could be due to the conservative nature of drug companies, and perhaps a concern about trivializing medicines and illness by associating them with entertainment. Or maybe, at a time when DTC is being so closely scrutinized, companies would just as soon keep whatever product placement marketing they're engaged in as quiet as possible.

Nonetheless, Frosch says the potential for pharma product-placement marketing remains, and the inclusion of drug names in scripts is, at present, poorly supervised. Drugs are a different kind of product, says Frosch, and promoting them through product placements requires new FDA guidelines.

Pharmaceutical product placements integrate brands into story lines and may be an evolution in the industry's focus on direct-to-consumer advertising. Although it is still uncommon, the potential for such marketing is present and warrants attention. Medications have a unique status as a product category, and policies need to be tailored accordingly.

ORIGINS

Product placement began in the 19th century. By the time Jules Verne ublished the adventure novel Around the World in Eighty Days(1873), his fame had led transport and shipping companies to lobby to be mentioned in the story. Whether Verne was actually paid to do so, however, remains unknown. Similarly, a painting by Eduoard Manet (1881-1882) shows a bar at the Folies Bergere with distinctive bottles placed at either end of the counter. The beer bottle is immediately recognisable as Bass beer. Manet’s motivations for including branded products in his painting are unknown; it may be that it simply added to the work’s authenticity, but on the other hand the artist may have received some payment in return for its inclusion.

Research reported by Jean-Marc Lehu (2007) suggests that films produced by Auguste and Louis Lumière in 1876 were made at the request of a representative of Lever Brothers in France. The films feature Sunlight soap, which may be the first recorded instance of paid product placement in film. This led to cinema becoming one of the earliest channels used for product placement.

Self-advertising: A German countess holds a copy of the magazine Die Woche in her hands. The photo appeared in 1902 in an issue of the magazine. (detail of the actual photograph)

With the arrival of photo-rich periodicals in the late 19th century, publishers found ways of lifting their paper's reputation by placing an actual copy of the magazine in photographs of prominent people. For example, the German magazine Die Woche in 1902 printed an article about a countess in her castle where she, in one of the photographs, holds a copy of the magazine in her hands.

Product placement was a common feature of many of the earliest actualities and cinematic attractions from the first ten years of cinema history.

During the next four decades, Harrison's Reports frequently cited cases of on-screen brand-name products. Harrison condemned the practice as harmful to movie theatres, and his editorials reflected his hostility towards product placement in films. Harrison's Reportspublished its first denunciation of that practice over Red Crown gasoline's appearance in The Garage (1920). Another editorial criticised the collaboration between the Corona Typewriter company and First National Pictures when a Corona typewriter appeared in several films in the mid-1920s including The Lost World (1925).

Recognisable brand names appeared in movies from cinema's earliest history. Before films were even narrative forms in the sense that they are recognized today, industrial concerns funded the making of what film scholar Tom Gunning described as "cinematic attractions", short films of one or two minutes. In the first decade or so of film (1895–1907) audiences attended films as "fairground attractions" interesting for their then-amazing visual effects. This format was better suited to product placement than narrative cinema. Gurevitch argued that early cinematic attractions have more in common with television advertisements in the 1950s than they do with traditional films. Gurevitch suggested that as a result, the relationship between cinema and advertising is intertwined, suggesting that cinema was in part the result of advertising and the economic advantage that it provided early film makers. Segrave detailed the industries that advertised in these early films.

Legal considerations

United States

Much of U.S. broadcast law pertaining to on-air product promotion dates to the payola scandals of 1950s broadcast radio. An investigation launched in November 1959 into allegations that some radio disc jockeys had accepted bribes in return for radio airplay ended with a US$2,500 fine for disc jockey Alan Freed (of WABC and WINS) for violating commercial bribery laws. On September 13, 1960, the U.S. government banned payola in broadcasting. Under 47 U.S.C. § 317 "All matter broadcast by any radio station for which money, service, or other valuable consideration is directly or indirectly paid, or promised to or charged or accepted by, the station so broadcasting, from any person, shall, at the time the same is so broadcast, be announced as paid for or furnished, as the case may be, by such person..." with similar and related provisions reflected in Federal Communications Commission regulations as 47 C.F.R. 73.1212.

These provisions have governed subsequent payola investigations, including a 2005 investigation into Sony BMG and other major record companies.

Often, a broadcaster claimed to have complied by placing an acknowledgement in an inconspicuous place, such as embedded within the credits. In 2005 U.S. Federal Communications Commission commissioner Jonathan Adelstein stated "if broadcasters and cable TV companies insist on further commercializing new and other shows alike, that is their business. But if they do so without disclosing it to the viewing public, that is payola, and that is the FCC's business."

United Kingdom

The 'PP' icon, introduced by Ofcomto identify programs on television which contain product placement.

In the United Kingdom, placement by commercial broadcasters was forbidden prior to 2011. On February 28, 2011, telecommunications regulator Ofcomlegalised placements in certain types of programming. A placement must be "editorially justified" and not place "undue prominence" on the product. Product placements are not allowed for products that cannot legally be advertised on television, including alcohol, baby milk, gambling products, medication or junk food. Placements are not allowed during children's, news, public affairs and religious programs. Additionally, broadcasters must disclose placements on-air by displaying a "PP" icon on-screen during the program for at least three seconds at the beginning, after every commercial break, and at the end. The first legal product placement on British television came during an episode of This Morning, for a Nestlé-produced coffee maker. As with all other advertising, the BBC is barred from using placements on its publicly funded services.

Extreme Examples

I, Robot offers placements for Converse, Ovaltine, Audi, FedEx, Dos Equis and JVC among others, all of them introduced within the film's first ten minutes. One moment includes a straightforward advertisement where Will Smith's character responds to a compliment about his shoes, to which he replies "Converse All-Stars, vintage 2004" (the year of the film's release). Audi created a special car for the film, the Audi RSQ. Surveys conducted in the US showed that the placements boosted the brand's image. The Audi RSQ appears for nine minutes, and other Audis also appear in the film. I, Robotwas ranked "the worst film for product placement" on a British site.

Demolition Man makes heavy mention of the only remaining restaurant chain being Taco Bell (in the U.S. release) or Pizza Hut (in the European release).

The Island features at least 35 individual products or brands, including cars, bottled water, shoes, credit cards, beer, ice cream, and a web search engine. In the movie's DVD Commentary track, director Michael Bay claims he added the advertisements for greater realism.

The 2006 comedy film Talladega Nights: The Ballad of Ricky Bobby parodied the large amount of sponsorship in NASCAR. For example, Ricky Bobby thanks baby Jesus for certain products during the dinner blessings, due to contractual obligations. In one race, he drives his car with a giant Fig Newtons sticker on his windshield, which obscures his vision. A scene where Ricky's and Jean Girard's cars go flipping for an excessively long time is interrupted by an Applebee's commercial (referencing NBC's use of commercial breaks during its own coverage). The character Jean Girard, a cultured French driver, is appropriately sponsored by Perrier mineral water.

Josie and the Pussycats contains placements in most of the shots. This appears to be done ironically, as the plot of the film revolves around subliminal messages in advertising. The film's general message can also be construed as an anti-consumerist one. The film neither sought nor received compensation for the placements.

The 2009 Star Trek, in a scene where young James Kirk drives and crashes a Chevrolet Corvette, he operates a Nokia touch-screen smartphone. Before running the car off the cliff while being chased by a hovering motorcycle cop, the distinct Nokia trademark ring tone can be heard. The Finnish phone maker offered Star Trek apps for its phones. The use of contemporary products was ridiculed, as the scene is set in the year 2255.

The 2013 Filipino film My Little Bossings attracted criticism for its extensive use of product placement. Reviewers panned the film for being "one long commercial", where advertisements for brands endorsed by the characters' actors are frequently interspersed into the film. Zig Marasigan of Rappler described the film's use of product endorsements as "some of the most distasteful examples of local product placement while no effort is made to weave them into the narrative." In a similar vein to early radio and television programs, sponsored programs in the Philippines are not uncommon, where children's programs like Tropang Potchi and Jollitown were produced on behalf of companies, prominently featuring products and related properties in the shows in question.

Viewer Response

In April 2009, fans of the television series Chuck responded to a placement by Subway restaurants with a grassroots effort to save the show from cancellation. The movement gained support from cast and crew, with series star Zachary Levi leading hundreds of fans to a Subway restaurant in Birmingham, United Kingdom.

Criticisms

Placement continues to grow, despite consumer groups such as Commercial Alert that object to the practise as "an affront to basic honesty". The group requested disclosure of all product-placement arrangements and notification before and during embedded advertisements. It justifies this to allow parents to protect easily influenced children.

In 2005, the Writers Guild of America, a trade union representing authors of television scripts, objected that its members were forced to produce disguised ad copy.

Some scholars argue that product placement may inherently affect the creativity and originality of movies as film producers may re-write scripts in order to incorporate products.Most typically, product placement and merchandise are most successful amongst specific genres of movies which may eventually limit the diversity of films.

Research

Effectiveness

As with most marketing tactics, product placement leads to explicit as well as implicit advertising effects. Explicit effects can be observed directly and are usually visible by higher recall scores. They are highly connected to the conscious mind. Implicit effects can be observed by a change in behavior – like a higher purchase intention.They are fully based on the subconscious mind. Implicit effects are more relevant for purchase decisions and therefore more valuable than explicit reactions.

Recall

Recall describes whether people can name a product after seeing it within the content. Research showed that there is a significant relationship between product placement and recall.

Attitude

Product placement also leads to changes in attitude towards the product or brand.

Purchase intention

A lot of research has shown a higher purchase intention as a result of product placement.

Subconscious Effects

Product placement affects the audience on a conscious, but also subconscious level. Science showed that there does not even need to be an explicit, conscious effect to activate subconscious effects. For example, product placement can lead to an exclusion of competing brands from the consideration set of the audience –

subconsciously. It is also hoped to bypass advertising defense reactions of consumers by focusing on the subconscious character of product placement.

Negative Effects

Under specific circumstances, product placement can lead to no or even negative effects. This usually happens if the product placement is too obvious, while the audience also feels it is being manipulated.

Placement Moderators

Congruence

The better the product placement fits the surrounding content, the better the implicit effectiveness (like attitude or purchase-intention) will be.

Audio Vs Visual

After viewing a Seinfeld episode with visual, auditory and audiovisual product placements, a recall task indicated that audiovisual product placements were recalled the best, visual product placements somewhat less and audio placements least. In a recognition test audiovisual was still remembered the best but audio placements were remembered second best and visual placements were remembered third best. As indicated, the type of placement that is most effective seems to vary depending on task, but audiovisual placements seem to be often the most effective. However, audiovisual product placements are not remembered best when there is more than one audiovisual placement at once, making it hard to remember each one. In case the placement is only on the audio level, advertisers must make sure it is very prominent to have any effect at all.

Character Attractiveness

People tended to like brand names that were paired with attractive faces more than those paired with unattractive faces. The more times a brand was paired with an attractive face, the more people liked it.

Product Prominence

Product placement perceived to disrupt a movie, especially when repeated, were found in one study to be counterproductive. Moderate repetition of subtle product placements did not increase people's feelings of distraction.

Products that are integrated within the plot of a movie are better recall, although not if more than one product is shown at a time. In one study placements connected to the story were recognized most often, products used by the main character were remembered less often and products in the background were remembered least often.

Placements were found more effective on a larger screen compared to on a smaller one. Also, products placed in the first half of a movie tend to be remembered better than products in the second half of a movie, which demonstrates the primacy effect.

Level of Involvement

High involvement with the program makes it easier for people to recognize the product placement. This can lead to positive effects, but might also lead to negative reactions. The same applies for high product category involvement.

Audience Demographics

Cultural attributes

Older research cited a difference between different cultural areas. For example, Australians, Austrians. and Germans tended to evaluate product placement more critically and show less positive reactions than Americans or people from certain Asian countries such as India.

Age

Children are usually more easily influenced than adults.

Sex

If the product is endorsed by a person, there are stronger priming effects if the audience is the same sex. Women tend to be influenced a little easier, but show more negative reactions when the product can be described as ethically questionable (e.g. alcohol).

Measurement

To measure the success of product placement, one first tracks the parameters of the placement itself, like the ease of identification, screen time, number of exposure(s), or association with a main character. That information is also often used to determine the price of a specific placement. Secondly, the effectiveness is measured using direct (for explicit memory effects) as well as indirect (for implicit memory effects) measurements.

Measurement of the Explicit Memory

Explicit effects are measured by recall or recognition tests. Subjects are asked to name the products that he or she noticed (free recall). This survey can be also aided by giving additional information like a specific product category. At recognition tests, a selection of products is shown to the interviewed person, who then needs to select the ones that he has seen before.

Measurement of the Implicit Memory

Implicit effects are measured in an indirect way by observing a change in behavior. This can be done by tracking the consideration set and buying behavior of people, measuring brain activities or using abstract indirect test settings like the word fragment or word stem completion test. The implicit association test (IAT) is also an applicable measurement tool.

Ethics

Many argue that product placement is ethically questionable, because it manipulates people against their will. A contrary view is, even if product placement is only perceived unconsciously, it is still evaluated by our mind. It cannot make people act against their beliefs. Most people also appreciate the fact that movies look more realistic with real brands and do not feel disturbed by the placements. Additionally, further research argues that product placement is not any different from other marketing tactics when it comes to ethics.

Sales Promotion

Sales Promotion is one of the elements of the promotional mix. (The primary elements in the promotional mix are advertising, personal selling, direct marketing and publicity/public relations). Sales promotion uses both media and non-media marketing communications for a pre-determined, limited time to increase consumer demand, stimulate market demand or improve product availability. Examples include contests, coupons, freebies, loss leaders, point of purchase displays, premiums, prizes, product samples, and rebates.

Sales promotions can be directed at either the customer, sales staff, or distribution channel members (such as retailers). Sales promotions targeted at the consumer are called consumer sales promotions. Sales promotions targeted at retailers and wholesaleare called trade sales promotions.

Sales promotion includes several communications activities that attempt to provide added value or incentives to consumers, wholesalers, retailers, or other organizational customers to stimulate immediate sales. These efforts can attempt to stimulate product interest, trial, or purchase. Examples of devices used in sales promotion include coupons, samples, premiums, point-of-purchase (POP) displays, contests, rebates, and sweepstakes.

Sales promotion is implemented to attract new customers, to hold present customers, to counteract competition, and to take advantage of opportunities that are revealed by market research. It is made up of activities, both outside and inside activities, to enhance company sales. Outside sales promotion activities include advertising, publicity, public relations activities, and special sales events. Inside sales promotion activities include window displays, product and promotional material display and promotional programs such as premium awards and contests.

Sale promotions often come in the form of discounts. Discounts impact the way consumers think and behave when shopping. The type of savings and its location can affect the way consumers view a product and affect their purchase decision. The two most common discounts are price discounts ("on sale items") and bonus packs ("bulk items"). Price discounts are the reduction of an original sale by a certain percentage while bonus packs are deals in which the consumer receives more for the original price. Many companies present different forms of discounts in advertisements, hoping to convince consumers to buy their products.

Sales Promotion: Definition

Sales promotion represents a variety of techniques used to stimulate the purchase of a product or brand. Sales promotion has a tactical, rather than strategic role in marketing communications and brand strategy, it is also a form of advertisement used within a short period of time. Researchers Farhangmehr and Brito, reviewed the definitions of sales promotions in marketing texts and journals and identified a set of common characteristics of sales promotion, including:

- Short-term effects and duration;
- Operates and influences only the last phase of the purchase process;
- Exhibits a secondary role in relation to other forms of marketing communication;
- Performs an accessory role regarding the products core benefits
- Is not a single technique, rather it is a set of techniques used for a specific purpose

Both manufacturers and retailers make extensive use of sales promotions. Retailer-sponsored sales promotions are directed at consumers. Manufacturers use two types of sales promotion, namely:

1. Consumer sales promotions: Sales promotions targeted at consumers or end-users and designed to stimulate the actual purchase
2. Trade promotions: Sales promotions targeted at trade, especially retailers, designed to increase sales to retailers, to carry the product or brand or to support the retailer in consumer-oriented promotions

Consumer Sales Promotion Types

Consumer sales promotions are short term techniques designed to achieve short term objectives, such as to stimulate a purchase, encourage store traffic or simply to build excitement for a product or brand. Traditional sales promotions techniques include:

- Price deal: A temporary reduction in the price, such as 50% off.
- Loyal Reward Program: Consumers collect points, miles, or credits for purchases and redeem them for rewards.
- Cents-off deal: Offers a brand at a lower price. Price reduction may be a percentage marked on the package.

- Price-pack/Bonus packs deal: The packaging offers a consumer a certain percentage more of the product for the same price (for example, 25 percent extra). This is another type of deal "in which customers are offered more of the product for the same price". For example, a sales company may offer their consumers a bonus pack in which they can receive two products for the price of one. In these scenarios, this bonus pack is framed as a gain because buyers believe that they are obtaining a free product. The purchase of a bonus pack, however, is not always beneficial for the consumer. Sometimes consumers will end up spending money on an item they would not normally buy had it not been in a bonus pack. As a result, items bought in a bonus pack are often wasted and is viewed as a "loss" for the consumer.
- Coupons: coupons have become a standard mechanism for sales promotions.
- Loss leader: the price of a popular product is temporarily reduced below cost in order to stimulate other profitable sales
- Free-standing insert (FSI): A coupon booklet is inserted into the local newspaper for delivery.
- Checkout dispensers: On checkout the customer is given a coupon based on products purchased.
- Mobile couponing: Coupons are available on a mobile phone. Consumers show the offer on a mobile phone to a salesperson for redemption.
- Online interactive promotion game: Consumers play an interactive game associated with the promoted product.
- Rebates: Consumers are offered money back if the receipt and barcode are mailed to the producer.
- Contests/sweepstakes/games: The consumer is automatically entered into the event by purchasing the product.
- Point-of-sale displays:-
- Aisle interrupter: A sign that juts into the aisle from the shelf.
- Dangler: A sign that sways when a consumer walks by it.
- Dump bin: A bin full of products dumped inside.
- Bidding portals: Getting prospects
- Glorifier: A small stage that elevates a product above other products.
- Wobbler: A sign that jiggles.
- Lipstick Board: A board on which messages are written in crayon.
- Necker: A coupon placed on the 'neck' of a bottle.

- YES unit: "your extra salesperson" is a pull-out fact sheet.
- Electroluminescent: Solar-powered, animated light in motion.
- Kids eat free specials: Offers a discount on the total dining bill by offering 1 free kids meal with each regular meal purchased.
- Sampling: Consumers get one sample for free, after their trial and then could decide whether to buy or not.

New technologies have provided a range of new opportunities for sales promotions. Loyalty cards, personal shopping assistants, electronic shelf labels, and electronic advertising displays allow for more personalised communications and more targeted information at the point of purchase. For example, shoppers may receive alerts for special offers when they approach a product in a specific aisle.

ONLINE DEALS VS. IN-STORE DEALS

There are different types of discounts available online versus in the stores. On-shelf couponing: Coupons are present at the shelf where the product is available. * On-line couponing: Coupons are available online. Consumers print them out and take them to the store.Although discounts can be found online and in stores, there is a different thought process when shopping in each location. For example, "online shoppers are more price-sensitive because of the readily available low search cost and direct price comparisons". Consumers can easily go to other websites and find better deals as opposed to physically going to various stores. In addition, buyers tend to refrain from purchasing bonus packs online because of the skepticism (of fraud and scams) that may come with the deal. Since "...bonus packs are more difficult than price discounts to process online, they are more difficult and effortful for the consumer to understand". For example, a buy-one-get-one-free deal on a website requires more work than the same bonus pack offered in a store. Online, consumers have to deal with payment processing, shipping and handling fees, and days waiting for the products' arrival, while in a store, the products are available without those additional steps and delays.

Trade sales Promotion Techniques

- Trade allowances: short term incentive offered to induce a retailer to stock up on a product.
- Dealer loader: An incentive given to induce a retailer to purchase and display a product.
- Trade contest: A contest to reward retailers that sell the most product.
- Point-of-purchase displays: Used to create the urge of "impulse" buying and selling your product on the spot.
- Training programs: dealer employees are trained in selling the product.
- Push money: also known as "spiffs". An extra commission paid to retail employees to push products.

Trade discounts (also called functional discounts): These are payments to distribution channel members for performing some function .

Retail Mechanics

Retailers have a stock number of retail 'mechanics' that they regularly roll out or rotate for new marketing initiatives.

- Buy x get y free a.k.a. BOGOF for Buy One Get One Free
- Three for two
- Buy a quantity for a lower price
- Get x% of discount on weekdays.
- Free gift with purchase

Consumer Thought Process

Meaningful Savings: Gain or Loss

Many discounts are designed to give consumers the perception of saving money when buying products, but not all discounted prices are viewed as favorable to buyers. Therefore, before making a purchase, consumers may weigh their options as either a gain or a loss to avoid the risk of losing money on a purchase. A "gain" view on a purchase results in chance taking. For example, if there is a buy-one-get-one-half-off discount that seems profitable, a shopper will buy the product. On the other hand, a "loss" viewpoint results in consumer aversion to taking any chances. For instance, consumers will pass on a buy-three-get-one-half-off discount if they believe they are not benefitting from the deal. Specifically, consumers will consider their options because "…the sensation of loss is 2.5 times greater than the sensation of gain for the same value".

Impulse Buying

Impulse buying results from consumers' failure to weigh their options before buying a product. Impulse buying is "any purchase that a shopper makes that has not been planned… [and is] sudden and immediate". For example, if a consumer has no intention of buying a product before entering a store, but purchases an item without any forethought, that is impulse buying. Product manufactures want to promote and encourage this instant purchase impulse in consumers. Buyers can be very quick to make purchases without thinking about the consequences when a product is perceived to be a good deal. Therefore, sales companies "increasingly implement promotional campaigns that will be effective in triggering consumer impulse buying behavior" to increase sales and profit.

COMPARING PRICES

Many consumers read left-to-right, and therefore, compare prices in the same manner. For example, if the price of a product is $93 and the sales price is $79, people will initially compare the left digits first (9 and 7) and notice the two digit difference. However, because of this habitual behavior, "consumers may perceive the ($14) difference between $93 and $79 as greater than the ($14) difference between $89 and $75". As a result, consumers often mistakenly believe they are receiving a better deal with the first set of prices based on the left digits solely. Because of that common misconception, companies capitalize on this sales pricing strategy more often than not to increase sales.

Right Digit Effect

The right digit effect focuses on the right digits of prices when the left digits are the same. In other words, prices like $45 and $42 force consumers to pay more attention to the right digits (the 2 and 5) to determine the discount received. This effect also "implies that consumers will perceive larger discounts for prices with small right digit endings, than for large right digit endings. For example, in a $32-to-$31 price reduction, consumers will believe to have received a greater deal than a $39-to-$38 price reduction. As a result, companies may use discounts with smaller right digits to mislead consumers into thinking they are receiving a better deal and increasing profit. However, consumers also are deceived by the infamous 9-ending prices. "The right digit effect [also] relates to consumers' tendency to identify 9-ending prices as sale (rather than regular) prices or to associate them with a discount. For example, a regular price of $199 is mistakenly viewed as a sale or discount by consumers. Sales companies most commonly use this approach because the misinterpretation of consumers usually results in an increase of sales and profit.

Framing Effect

The Framing Effect is "the phenomenon that occurs when there is a change in an individual's preference between two or more alternatives caused by the way the problem is presented". In other words, the format in which something is presented will affect a person's viewpoint. This theory consists of three subcategories: risky choice framing, attribute framing and goal framing. Risky choice framing references back to the gain-or-loss thought processes of consumers. Consumers will take chances if the circumstance is profitable for them and avoid chance-taking if it is not. Attribute framing deals with one key phrase or feature of a price discount that is emphasized to inspire consumer shopping.For example, the terms "free" and "better" are used commonly to lure in shoppers to buy a product. Goal framing places pressure on buyers to act hastily or face the consequences of missing out on a definite price reduction. A "limited time only" (LTO) deal, for example, attempts to motivate buyers to make a purchase quickly, or buy on impulse, before the time runs out.

Outside Forces

Although there are aspects that can determine a consumer's shopping behavior, there are many outside factors that can influence the shoppers' decision in making a purchase. For example, even though a product's price is discounted, the quality of that product may dissuade the consumer from buying the item. If the product has poor customer reviews or has a short "life span," shoppers will view that purchase as a loss and avoid taking a chance on it. A product can also be viewed negatively because of consumers' past experiences and expectations. For example, if the size of a product is misleading, buyers will not want to buy it. An item advertised as "huge," but is only one inch tall, will ward off consumers. Also, "the effects of personal characteristics, such as consumers' gender, subjective norms, and impulsivity" can also affect a consumer's purchase intentions. For example, a female will, generally, purchase a cosmetic product more often than a male. In addition, "some...shoppers may be unable to buy [a product]...because of financial constraints". Neither a discounted price nor a bonus pack has the ability to entice consumers if they cannot afford the product.

Political issues

Sales promotions have traditionally been heavily regulated in many advanced industrial nations, with the notable exception of the United States. For example, the United Kingdomformerly operated under a resale price maintenance regime in which manufacturers could legally dictate the minimum resale price for virtually all goods; this practice was abolished in 1964.

Most European countries also have controls on the scheduling and permissible types of sales promotions, as they are regarded in those countries as bordering upon unfair business practices. Germany is notorious for having the most strict regulations. Famous examples include the car wash that was barred from giving free car washes to regular customers and a baker who could not give a free cloth bag to customers who bought more than 10 rolls.

10

Online Advertising of Pharma Products

Form of marketing and advertising which uses the Internet to deliver promotional marketing messages to consumers. Consumers view online advertising as an unwanted distraction with few benefits and have increasingly turned to ad blocking for a variety of reasons. When software is used to do the purchasing, it is known as programmatic advertising.

It includes email marketing, search engine marketing (SEM), social media marketing, many types of display advertising (including web banner advertising), and mobile advertising. Like other advertising media, online advertising frequently involves both a publisher, who integrates advertisements into its online content, and an advertiser, who provides the advertisements to be displayed on the publisher's content. Other potential participants include advertising agencies who help generate and place the ad copy, an ad server which technologically delivers the ad and tracks statistics, and advertising affiliates who do independent promotional work for the advertiser.

In 2016, Internet advertising revenues in the United States surpassed those of cable television and broadcast television. In 2017, Internet advertising revenues in the United States totaled $83.0 billion, a 14% increase over the $72.50 billion in revenues in 2016.

Many common online advertising practices are controversial and increasingly subject to regulation. Online ad revenues may not adequately replace other publishers' revenue streams. Declining ad revenue has led some publishers to place their content behind paywalls.

Digital has already transformed the pharma and healthcare industry in many ways such as greater levels of transparency, patient communication and drug development.

In addition, due to its unrivalled cost-effectiveness, digital marketing strategies offer a variety of meaningful ways to connect and treat prospective clients and customers.

In this article, we explore the key trends and tactics that will help marketers in the pharma industry to use digital marketing to promote, engage and grow.

Pharmaceutical Marketing: The Internet impact

Faced with rising costs, shortened product lifecycles and an increasing reliance on blockbuster drugs, pharma companies are turning towards innovative marketing campaigns to reach an increasingly demanding consumer audience. Offering particular potential, online solutions are being introduced to establish profitable interactions with large numbers of consumers across multiple channels. The Market Brief 'Pharmaceutical Campaign Management' looks at the major factors that are currently shaping pharmaceutical marketing activities and examines a recent promotional campaign undertaken by a pharmaceutical company to illustrate the use of online and offline marketing. The brief moves on to look at the evolving structure of marketing campaigns, from traditional offline channels such as television through to customer relationship marketing and intelligent customer care.

The Future Decoded section examines the steps that pharmaceutical companies should be taking in order to incorporate campaign management into their marketing strategies over the next five years. New strategies needed Pharmaceutical companies are conservative in nature. They have developed tried-and-tested promotional strategies that have proven results. However, the rising costs of drug development and shortened drug lifecycles means that companies must examine new ways of creating new and innovative promotional strategies to maximize the revenue potential for each drug. The cost and limited success of traditional marketing campaigns has been the major subject to drive alternative marketing strategies. Drug companies are also having to look at additional methods to find media exposure because the market is becoming increasing competitive. The Internet is being recognized as another initiative that can bring the competitive edge. The current pharmaceutical marketing landscape is being driven by a number of changes, including changes in direct-to-consumer (DTC) advertising and the growth in consumer Internet use. In addition to the traditional marketing channels such as television and radio, pharmaceutical companies are using a new set of marketing channels to reach a large number of targeted consumers. Direct marketing is increasingly valuable and the Internet provides the means to reach consumers.

Online possibilities The Internet has many of the qualities of traditional media: it can provide the in-depth content seen in print advertising, the real-time impact of television, the immediate response of direct mail and the mass reach of outdoor advertising. With the rapid growth of online marketing, many Internet-based campaigns have often been added on to existing campaigns. Television adverts will often refer consumers to a disease or drug website, but that is often where the relationship stops. The online medium appears to be playing catch-up in prescription drug advertising, although this gap will reduce with time and experience. The Internet has provided pharmaceutical companies with further opportunities to carry out 'one-shot' marketing campaigns through website sponsorship and banners. Although consumer responses can be measured, for example through tracking the click-through rates, there is no clear measure of their effectiveness. The Internet is however, not without its challenges and is unlikely to replace direct mail or, indeed, any other channel completely. Furthermore, a significant proportion of the population do not use the Internet and due to the inverse relationship between age and Internet use this is particularly applicable for age-related therapeutic areas. Conventional marketing here to stay Conventional marketing tools will continue to be used because the leading drug makers are particularly keen to utilize any advertising methods that directly influence physicians.

The position of the doctor remains hugely significant. The FDA approves drugs for specific indications thereby only allowing a pharma company to promote the drug in that area. A physician however, can legally prescribe any medication for any use. It is therefore unsurprising that pharmaceutical organizations go to great lengths to influence medical opinion Pharmaceutical Reps act as the main method of contacting primary-care physician In a promotional activity known as 'detailing'. The importance of this endeavor is reflected by the size of sales forces at the major drug companies. In an article sponsored by the BlueCross BlueShield Association called "Getting Doctors to Say Yes to Drugs" the top companies were found to have an average of 4,000 representatives to sell to physicians plus 850 reps for specialists supported by an average budget of $875 million. Attention to eDetail Pharmaceutical sales and marketing teams can nevertheless use the Internet to interact with their direct customer base, the healthcare profession. eDetailing is essentially the use of the Internet to promote, or detail, a product to a physician, providing them with comprehensive information on new drugs or products, including clinical trial data, prescribing information and marketing materials.

Interactive websites are able to offer information detailing products in an engaging format that is available to physicians at any time. With cost significantly reduced eDetailing via interactive websites and devices can be an ideal way of raising physician awareness of new products and of increasing prescription rates. The use if the Internet in pharmaceutical marketing will also increase when return on investment (ROI) can be measured more accurately. Pharmaceutical companies need to see evidence of ROI and are concerned by both the cost and size of executing large-scale campaign management strategies. To date, online marketing channels such as Internet websites and email marketing campaigns have been viewed as 'add-on' features to existing campaigns rather than as integral components. But with increasing evidence showing the effectiveness of online marketing combined with reduced costs, the Internet looks set to become a more fundamental aspect of pharmaceutical marketing strategy.

1) Value-Driven Content Creation

One of the most significant transformations seen by digital's influence on the pharma industry is the fact that pharmaceutical companies are no longer the sole gatekeepers or providers of the information surrounding their treatments or products.

Through online communities, mobile applications and a wealth of web content, people now have wide access to a range of pharma-based insights. By creating targeted, value-driven branded content that offers prospective or current patients insight into relevant information, you can grow your audience, significantly.

By providing answers to common patient pain points in an inspiring, engaging way alongside demonstrating transparency, you will grow your audience while fostering trust and positioning your brand as a thought-leader.

As an international healthcare brand, Johnson & Johnson are renowned for their wealth of inspiring content marketing initiatives but of all its campaigns, its 'Care Inspires Care' campaign is perhaps the most inspiring.

Boasting the perfect mix of value-driven, blog content, emotive messaging, social media posts, and eye-grabbing visuals, this particular campaign honed in on the importance of caring for one another. By prompting people to share their random acts of care through Facebook and supporting the campaign with a host of share-worthy content, the brand encouraged a total of 26 million acts of care - and counting.

In early days of the Internet, online advertising was mostly prohibited. For example, two of the predecessor networks to the Internet, ARPANET and NSFNet, had "acceptable use policies" that banned network "use for commercial activities by for-profit institutions". The NSFNet began phasing out its commercial use ban in 1991.

Email

The first widely publicized example of online advertising was conducted via electronic mail. On 3 May 1978, a marketer from DEC (Digital Equipment Corporation), Gary Thuerk, sent an email to most of the ARPANET's American west coast users, advertising an open house for a new model of a DEC computer. Despite the prevailing acceptable use policies, electronic mail marketing rapidly expanded and eventually became known as "spam."

The first known large-scale non-commercial spam message was sent on 18 January 1994 by an Andrews University system administrator, by cross-posting a religious message to all USENET newsgroups. In January 1994 Mark Eberra started the first email marketing company for opt in email list under the domain

Insideconnect.com. He also started the Direct Email Marketing Association to help stop unwanted email and prevent spam.

Four months later, Laurence Canter and Martha Siegel, partners in a law firm, broadly promoted their legal services in a USENET posting titled "Green Card Lottery – Final One?"Canter and Siegel's Green Card USENET spam raised the profile of online advertising, stimulating widespread interest in advertising via both Usenet and traditional email. More recently, spam has evolved into a more industrial operation, where spammers use armies of virus-infected computers (botnets) to send spam remotely.

Display Ads

Online banner advertising began in the early 1990s as page owners sought additional revenue streams to support their content. Commercial online service Prodigy displayed banners at the bottom of the screen to promote Sears products. The first clickable web ad was sold by Global Network Navigator in 1993 to a Silicon Valley law firm. In 1994, web banner advertising became mainstream when HotWired, the online component of Wired Magazine, sold banner ads to AT&T and other companies. The first AT&T ad on HotWired had a 44% click-through rate, and instead of directing clickers to AT&T's website, the ad linked to an online tour of seven of the world's most acclaimed art museums.

Search Ads

GoTo.com (renamed Overture in 2001, and acquired by Yahoo! in 2003) created the first search advertising keyword auction in 1998. Google launched its "AdWords" search advertising program in 2000 and introduced quality-based ranking allocation in 2002, which sorts search advertisements by a combination of bid price and searchers' likeliness to click on the ads.

Recent Trends

More recently, companies have sought to merge their advertising messages into editorial content or valuable services. Examples include Red Bull's Red Bull Media House streaming Felix Baumgartner's jump from space online, Coca-Cola's online magazines, and Nike's free applications for performance tracking. Advertisers are also embracing social media and mobile advertising; mobile ad spending has grown 90% each year from 2010 to 2013.

Example of Display Advertisingfeaturing Geotargeting

Display advertising conveys its advertising message visually using text, logos, animations, videos, photographs, or other graphics. Display advertisers frequently target users with particular traits to increase the ads' effect. Online advertisers (typically through their ad servers) often use cookies, which are unique identifiers of specific computers, to decide which ads to serve to a particular consumer. Cookies can track whether a user left a page without buying anything, so the advertiser can later retarget the user with ads from the site the user visited.

As advertisers collect data across multiple external websites about a user's online activity, they can create a detailed profile of the user's interests to deliver even more targeted advertising. This aggregation of data is called behavioral targeting. Advertisers can also target their audience by using contextual to deliver display ads related to the content of the web page where the ads appear. Retargeting, behavioral targeting, and contextual advertising all are designed to increase an advertiser's return on investment, or ROI, over untargeted ads.

Advertisers may also deliver ads based on a user's suspected geography through geotargeting. A user's IP address communicates some geographic information (at minimum, the user's country or general region). The geographic information from an IP can be supplemented and refined with other proxies or information to narrow the range of possible locations. For example, with mobile devices, advertisers can sometimes use a phone's GPS receiver or the location of nearby mobile towers. Cookies and other persistent data on a user's machine may provide help narrowing a user's location further.

Web banner Advertising

Web banners or banner ads typically are graphical ads displayed within a web page. Many banner ads are delivered by a central ad server.

Banner ads can use rich media to incorporate video, audio, animations, buttons, forms, or other interactive elements using Java applets, HTML5, Adobe Flash, and other programs.

Frame ad (Traditional Banner)

Frame ads were the first form of web banners. The colloquial usage of "banner ads" often refers to traditional frame ads. Website publishers incorporate frame ads by setting aside a particular space on the web page. The Interactive Advertising Bureau's Ad Unit Guidelines proposes standardized pixel dimensions for ad units.

POP-UPS/POP-UNDERS

A pop-up ad is displayed in a new web browser window that opens above a website visitor's initial browser window. A pop-under ad opens a new browser window under a website visitor's initial browser window. Pop-under ads and similar technologies are now advised against by online authorities such as Google, who state that they "do not condone this practice".

Floating Ad

A floating ad, or overlay ad, is a type of rich media advertisement that appears superimposed over the requested website's content. Floating ads may disappear or become less obtrusive after a preset time period.

Expanding Ad

An expanding ad is a rich media frame ad that changes dimensions upon a predefined condition, such as a preset amount of time a visitor spends on a webpage, the user's click on the ad, or the user's mouse movement over the ad. Expanding ads allow advertisers to fit more information into a restricted ad space.

Trick Banners

A trick banner is a banner ad where the ad copy imitates some screen element users commonly encounter, such as an operating system message or popular application message, to induce ad clicks. Trick banners typically do not mention the advertiser in the initial ad, and thus they are a form of bait-and-switch. Trick banners commonly attract a higher-than-average click-through rate, but tricked users may resent the advertiser for deceiving them.

News Feed Ads

"News Feed Ads", also called "Sponsored Stories", "Boosted Posts", typically exist on social media platforms that offer a steady stream of information updates ("news feed") in regulated formats (i.e. in similar sized small boxes with a uniform style). Those advertisements are intertwined with non-promoted news that the users are reading through. Those advertisements can be of any content, such as promoting a website, a fan page, an app, or a product.

Some examples are: Facebook's "Sponsored Stories", LinkedIn's "Sponsored Updates", and Twitter's "Promoted Tweets".

This display ads format falls into its own category because unlike banner ads which are quite distinguishable, News Feed Ads' format blends well into non-paid news updates. This format of online advertisement yields much higher click-through rates than traditional display ads.

Display Advertising Process Overview

The process by which online advertising is displayed can involve many parties. In the simplest case, the website publisher selects and serves the ads. Publishers which operate their own advertising departments may use this method.

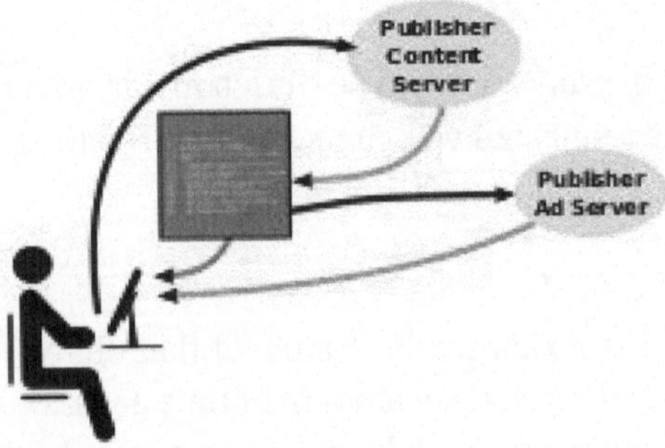

Online advertising serving process - simple publisher case

The ads may be outsourced to an advertising agency under contract with the publisher, and served from the advertising agency's servers.

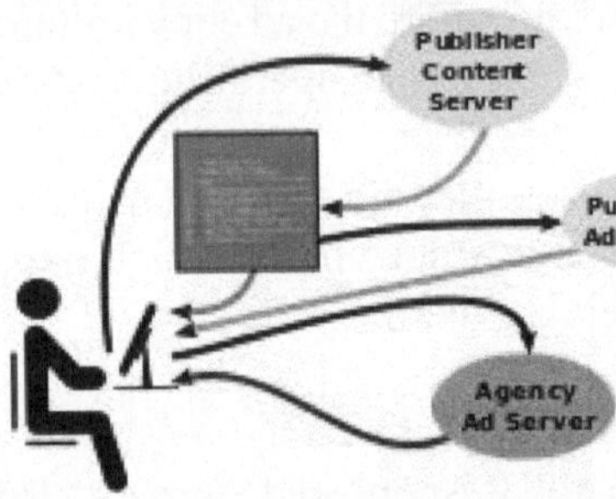

Online advertising serving process using an ad agency

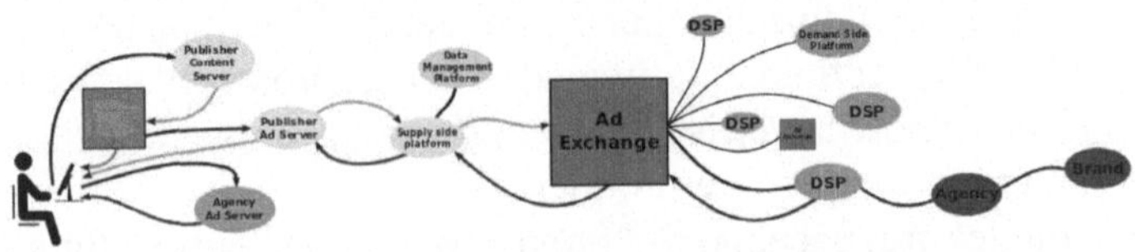

Online advertising serving process using online bidding

Alternatively, ad space may be offered for sale in a bidding market using an ad exchange and real-time bidding. This involves many parties interacting automatically in real time. In response to a request from the user's browser, the publisher content server sends the web page content to the user's browser over the Internet. The page does not yet contain ads, but contains links which cause the user's browser to connect to the publisher ad server to request that the spaces left for ads be filled in with ads. Information identifying the user, such as cookiesand the page being viewed, is transmitted to the publisher ad server.

The publisher ad server then communicates with a supply-side platform server. The publisher is offering ad space for sale, so they are considered the supplier. The supply side platform also receives the user's identifying information, which it sends to a data management platform. At the data management platform, the user's identifying information is used to look up demographic information, previous purchases, and other information of interest to advertisers.

Broadly speaking, there are three types of data obtained through such a data management platform:

First party data refers to the data retrieved from customer relationship management (CRM) platforms, in addition to website and paid media content or cross-platform data. This can include data from customer behaviors, actions or interests.

Second party data refers to an amalgamation of statistics related to cookie pools on external publications and platforms. The data is provided directly from the source (adservers, hosted solutions for social or an analytics platform). It is also possible to negotiate a deal with a particular publisher to secure specific data points or audiences.

Third party data is sourced from external providers and often aggregated from numerous websites. Businesses sell third-party data and are able to share this via an array of distribution avenues.

This customer information is combined and returned to the supply side platform, which can now package up the offer of ad space along with information about the user who will view it. The supply side platform sends that offer to an ad exchange.

The ad exchange puts the offer out for bid to demand-side platforms. Demand side platforms act on behalf of ad agencies, who sell ads which advertise brands. Demand side platforms thus have ads ready to display, and are searching for users to view them. Bidders get the information about the user ready to view the ad, and decide, based on that information, how much to offer to buy the ad space. According to the Internet Advertising Bureau, a demand side platform has 10 milliseconds to respond to an offer. The ad exchange picks the winning bid and informs both parties.

The ad exchange then passes the link to the ad back through the supply side platform and the publisher's ad server to the user's browser, which then requests the ad content from the agency's ad server. The ad agency can thus confirm that the ad was delivered to the browser.

This is simplified, according to the IAB. Exchanges may try to unload unsold ("remnant") space at low prices through other exchanges. Some agencies maintain semi-permanent pre-cached bids with ad exchanges, and those may be examined before going out to additional demand side platforms for bids. The process for mobile advertising is different and may involve mobile carriers and handset software manufacturers.

Interstitial

An interstitial ad displays before a user can access requested content, sometimes while the user is waiting for the content to load. Interstitial ads are a form of interruption marketing.

Text Ads

A text ad displays text-based hyperlinks. Text-based ads may display separately from a web page's primary content, or they can be embedded by hyperlinking individual words or phrases to advertiser's websites. Text ads may also be delivered through email marketing or text message marketing. Text-based ads often render faster than graphical ads and can be harder for ad-blocking software to block.

Search Engine Marketing (SEM)

Search engine marketing, or SEM, is designed to increase a website's visibility in search engine results pages (SERPs). Search engines provide sponsored results and organic (non-sponsored) results based on a web searcher's query. Search engines often employ visual cues to differentiate sponsored results from organic results. Search engine marketing includes all of an advertiser's actions to make a website's listing more prominent for topical keywords.

Search Engine Optimization (SEO)

Search engine optimization, or SEO, attempts to improve a website's organic search rankings in SERPs by increasing the website content's relevance to search terms. Search engines regularly update their algorithms to penalize poor quality sites that try to game their rankings, making optimization a moving target for advertisers. Many vendors offer SEO services.

Sponsored Search

Sponsored search (also called sponsored links, search ads, or paid search) allows advertisers to be included in the sponsored results of a search for selected keywords. Search ads are often sold via real-time auctions, where advertisers bid on keywords. In addition to setting a maximum price per keyword, bids may include time, language, geographical, and other constraints. Search engines originally sold listings in order of highest bids. Modern search engines rank sponsored listings based on a combination of bid price, expected click-through rate, keyword relevancy and site quality.

Social Media Marketing

Social media marketing is commercial promotion conducted through social media websites. Many companies promote their products by posting frequent updates and providing special offers through their social media profiles.

Mobile Advertising

Mobile advertising is ad copy delivered through wireless mobile devices such as smartphones, feature phones, or tablet computers. Mobile advertising may take the form of static or rich media display ads, SMS (Short Message Service) or MMS (Multimedia Messaging Service) ads, mobile search ads, advertising within mobile websites, or ads within mobile applications or games (such as interstitial ads, "advergaming," or application sponsorship). Industry groups such as the Mobile Marketing Association have attempted to standardize mobile ad unit specifications, similar to the IAB's efforts for general online advertising.

Mobile advertising is growing rapidly for several reasons. There are more mobile devices in the field, connectivity speeds have improved (which, among other things, allows for richer media ads to be served quickly), screen resolutions have advanced, mobile publishers are becoming more sophisticated about incorporating ads, and consumers are using mobile devices more extensively. The Interactive Advertising Bureau predicts continued growth in mobile advertising with the adoption of location-based targeting and other technological features not available or relevant on personal computers. In July 2014 Facebook reported advertising revenue for the June 2014 quarter of $2.68 billion, an increase of 67 percent over the second quarter of 2013. Of that, mobile advertising revenue accounted for around 62 percent, an increase of 41 percent on the previous year.

Email Advertising

Email advertising is ad copy comprising an entire email or a portion of an email message. Email marketing may be unsolicited, in which case the sender may give the recipient an option to opt out of future emails, or it may be sent with the recipient's prior consent (opt-in).

Chat Advertising

As opposed to static messaging, chat advertising refers to real time messages dropped to users on certain sites. This is done by the usage of live chat software or tracking applications installed within certain websites with the operating personnel behind the site often dropping adverts on the traffic surfing around the sites. In reality this is a subset of the email advertising but different because of its time window.

Online Classified Advertising

Online classified advertising is advertising posted online in a categorical listing of specific products or services. Examples include online job boards, online real estate listings, automotive listings, online yellow pages, and online auction-based listings. Craigslist and eBay are two prominent providers of online classified listings.

Adware

Adware is software that, once installed, automatically displays advertisements on a user's computer. The ads may appear in the software itself, integrated into web pages visited by the user, or in pop-ups/pop-unders. Adware installed without the user's permission is a type of malware.

Affiliate Marketing

Affiliate marketing occurs when advertisers organize third parties to generate potential customers for them. Third-party affiliates receive payment based on sales generated through their promotion. Affiliate marketers generate traffic to offers from affiliate networks, and when the desired action is taken by the visitor, the affiliate earns a commission. These desired actions can be an email submission, a phone call, filling out an online form, or an online order being completed.

Content Marketing

Content marketing is any marketing that involves the creation and sharing of media and publishing content in order to acquire and retain customers. This information can be presented in a variety of formats, including blogs, news, video, white papers, e-books, infographics, case studies, how-to guides and more. Considering that most marketing involves some form of published media, it is almost (though not entirely) redundant to call 'content marketing' anything other than simply 'marketing'. There are, of course, other forms of marketing (in-person marketing, telephone-based marketing, word of mouth marketing, etc.) where the label is more useful for identifying the type of marketing. However, even these are usually merely presenting content that they are marketing as information in a way that is different from traditional print, radio, TV, film, email, or web media.

Online Marketing Platform

Online marketing platform (OMP) is an integrated web-based platform that combines the benefits of a business directory, local search engine, search engine optimisation (SEO) tool, customer relationship management (CRM) package and content management system (CMS). Ebay and Amazon are used as online marketing and logistics management platforms. On Facebook, Twitter, YouTube, Pinterest, LinkedIn, and other Social Media, retail online marketing is also used. Online business marketing platforms such as Marketo, Aprimo, MarketBright and Pardot have been bought by major IT companies (Eloqua-Oracle, Neolane-Adobe and Unica-IBM).

Unlike television marketing in which Neilsen TV Ratings can be relied upon for viewing metrics, online advertisers do not have an independent party to verify viewing claims made by the big online platforms.

Compensation Methods

Advertisers and publishers use a wide range of payment calculation methods. In 2012, advertisers calculated 32% of online advertising transactions on a cost-per-impression basis, 66% on customer performance (e.g. cost per click or cost per acquisition), and 2% on hybrids of impression and performance methods.

CPM (Cost Per Mille)

Cost per mille, often abbreviated to CPM, means that advertisers pay for every thousand displays of their message to potential customers (mille is the Latin word for thousand). In the online context, ad displays are usually called "impressions." Definitions of an "impression" vary among publishers, and some impressions may not be charged because they don't represent a new exposure to an actual customer. Advertisers can use technologies such as web bugs to verify if an impression is actually delivered.

Publishers use a variety of techniques to increase page views, such as dividing content across multiple pages, repurposing someone else's content, using sensational titles, or publishing tabloid or sexual content.

CPM advertising is susceptible to "impression fraud," and advertisers who want visitors to their sites may not find per-impression payments a good proxy for the results they desire.

CPC (Cost Per Click)

CPC (Cost Per Click) or PPC (Pay per click) means advertisers pay each time a user clicks on the ad. CPC advertising works well when advertisers want visitors to their sites, but it's a less accurate measurement for advertisers looking to build brand awareness. CPC's market share has grown each year since its introduction, eclipsing CPM to dominate two-thirds of all online advertising compensation methods.

Like impressions, not all recorded clicks are valuable to advertisers. GoldSpot Media reported that up to 50% of clicks on static mobile banner ads are accidental and resulted in redirected visitors leaving the new site immediately.

CPE (Cost Per Engagement)

Cost per engagement aims to track not just that an ad unit loaded on the page (i.e., an impression was served), but also that the viewer actually saw and/or interacted with the ad.

CPV (Cost Per view)

Cost per view video advertising. Both Google and TubeMogul endorsed this standardized CPV metric to the IAB's (Interactive Advertising Bureau) Digital Video Committee, and it's garnering a notable amount of industry support. CPV is the primary benchmark used in YouTube Advertising Campaigns, as part of Google's AdWords platform.

CPI (cost per install)

The CPI compensation method is specific to mobile applications and mobile advertising. In CPI ad campaigns brands are charged a fixed of bid rate only when the application was installed.

Attribution of ad value

In marketing, "attribution" is the measurement of effectiveness of particular ads in a consumer's ultimate decision to purchase. Multiple ad impressions may lead to a consumer "click" or other action. A single action may lead to revenue being paid to multiple ad space sellers.

Other performance-based compensation

CPA (Cost Per Action or Cost Per Acquisition) or PPP (Pay Per Performance) advertising means the advertiser pays for the number of users who perform a desired activity, such as completing a purchase or filling out a registration form. Performance-based compensation can also incorporate revenue sharing, where publishers earn a percentage of the advertiser's profits made as a result of the ad. Performance-based compensation shifts the risk of failed advertising onto publishers.

Fixed Cost

Fixed cost compensation means advertisers pay a fixed cost for delivery of ads online, usually over a specified time period, irrespective of the ad's visibility or users' response to it. One examples is CPD (cost per day) where advertisers pay a fixed cost for publishing an ad for a day irrespective of impressions served or clicks.

BENEFITS OF ONLINE ADVERTISING

Cost

The low costs of electronic communication reduce the cost of displaying online advertisements compared to offline ads. Online advertising, and in particular social media, provides a low-cost means for advertisers to engage with large established communities. Advertising online offers better returns than in other media.

Measurability

Online advertisers can collect data on their ads' effectiveness, such as the size of the potential audience or actual audience response, how a visitor reached their advertisement, whether the advertisement resulted in a sale, and whether an ad actually loaded within a visitor's view. This helps online advertisers improve their ad campaigns over time.

Formatting

Advertisers have a wide variety of ways of presenting their promotional messages, including the ability to convey images, video, audio, and links. Unlike many offline ads, online ads also can be interactive. For example, some ads let users input queries or let users follow the advertiser on social media. Online ads can even incorporate games.

Targeting

Publishers can offer advertisers the ability to reach customizable and narrow market segments for targeted advertising. Online advertising may use geo-targeting to display relevant advertisements to the user's geography. Advertisers can customize each individual ad to a particular user based on the user's previous preferences. Advertisers can also track whether a visitor has already seen a particular ad in order to reduce unwanted repetitious exposures and provide adequate time gaps between exposures.

Coverage

Online advertising can reach nearly every global market, and online advertising influences offline sales.

Speed

Once ad design is complete, online ads can be deployed immediately. The delivery of online ads does not need to be linked to the publisher's publication schedule. Furthermore, online advertisers can modify or replace ad copy more rapidly than their offline counterparts.

Concerns

Security concerns

According to a US Senate investigation, the current state of online advertising endangers the security and privacy of users.

Banner blindness

Eye-tracking studies have shown that Internet users often ignore web page zones likely to contain display ads (sometimes called "banner blindness"), and this problem is worse online than in offline media. On the other hand, studies suggest that even those ads "ignored" by the users may influence the user subconsciously.

Fraud on the advertiser

There are numerous ways that advertisers can be overcharged for their advertising. For example, click fraud occurs when a publisher or third parties click (manually or through automated means) on a CPC ad with no legitimate buying intent. For example, click fraud can occur when a competitor clicks on ads to deplete its rival's advertising budget, or when publishers attempt to manufacture revenue.

Click fraud is especially associated with pornography sites. In 2011, certain scamming porn websites launched dozens of hidden pages on each visitor's computer, forcing the visitor's computer to click on hundreds of paid links without the visitor's knowledge.

As with offline publications, online impression fraud can occur when publishers overstate the number of ad impressions they have delivered to their advertisers. To combat impression fraud, several publishing and advertising industry associations are developing ways to count online impressions credibly.

TECHNOLOGICAL VARIATIONS

Heterogeneous Clients

Because users have different operating systems, web browsers and computer hardware (including mobile devices and different screen sizes), online ads may appear to users differently from how the advertiser intended, or the ads may not display properly at all. A 2012 comScore study revealed that, on average, 31% of ads were not "in-view" when rendered, meaning they never had an opportunity to be seen. Rich media ads create even greater compatibility problems, as some developers may use competing (and exclusive) software to render the ads (see e.g. Comparison of HTML 5 and Flash).

Furthermore, advertisers may encounter legal problems if legally required information doesn't actually display to users, even if that failure is due to technological heterogeneity. In the United States, the FTC has released a set of guidelines indicating that it's the advertisers' responsibility to ensure the ads display any required disclosures or disclaimers, irrespective of the users' technology.

Ad Blocking

Ad blocking, or ad filtering, means the ads do not appear to the user because the user uses technology to screen out ads. Many browsers block unsolicited pop-up ads by default.Other software programs or browser add-ons may also block the loading of ads, or block elements on a page with behaviors characteristic of ads (e.g. HTML autoplay of both audio and video). Approximately 9% of all online page views come from browsers with ad-blocking software installed, and some publishers have 40%+ of their visitors using ad-blockers.

Anti-targeting Technologies

Some web browsers offer privacy modes where users can hide information about themselves from publishers and advertisers. Among other consequences, advertisers can't use cookies to serve targeted ads to private browsers. Most major browsers have incorporated Do Not Track options into their browser headers, but the regulations currently are only enforced by the honor system.

PRIVACY CONCERNS

The collection of user information by publishers and advertisers has raised consumer concerns about their privacy. Sixty percent of Internet users would use Do Not Track technology to block all collection of information if given an opportunity. Over half of all Google and Facebook users are concerned about their privacy when using Google and Facebook, according to Gallup.

Many consumers have reservations about online behavioral targeting. By tracking users' online activities, advertisers are able to understand consumers quite well. Advertisers often use technology, such as web bugs and respawning cookies, to maximizing their abilities to track consumers. According to a 2011 survey conducted by Harris Interactive, over half of Internet users had a negative impression of online behavioral advertising, and forty percent feared that their personally-identifiable information had been shared with advertisers without their consent. Consumers can be especially troubled by advertisers targeting them based on sensitive information, such as financial or health status.Furthermore, some advertisers attach the MAC address of users' devices to their 'demographic profiles' so they can be retargeted (regardless of the accuracy of the profile) even if the user clears their cookies and browsing history.

Trustworthiness of Advertisers

Scammers can take advantage of consumers' difficulties verifying an online persona's identity, leading to artifices like phishing (where scam emails look identical to those from a well-known brand owner) and confidence schemes like the Nigerian "419" scam. The Internet Crime Complaint Center received 289,874 complaints in 2012, totaling over half a billion dollars in losses, most of which originated with scam ads.

Consumers also face malware risks, i.e. malvertising, when interacting with online advertising. Cisco's 2013 Annual Security Report revealed that clicking on ads was 182 times more likely to install a virus on a user's computer than surfing the Internet for porn. For example, in August 2014 Yahoo's advertising network reportedly saw cases of infection of a variant of Cryptolocker ransomware.

Spam

The Internet's low cost of disseminating advertising contributes to spam, especially by large-scale spammers. Numerous efforts have been undertaken to combat spam, ranging from blacklists to regulatorily-required labeling to content filters, but most of those efforts have adverse collateral effects, such as mistaken filtering.

Regulation

In general, consumer protection laws apply equally to online and offline activities. However, there are questions over which jurisdiction's laws apply and which regulatory agencies have enforcement authority over transborder activity.

As with offline advertising, industry participants have undertaken numerous efforts to self-regulate and develop industry standards or codes of conduct. Several United States advertising industry organizations jointly published Self-Regulatory Principles for Online Behavioral Advertising based on standards proposed by the FTC in 2009. European ad associations published a similar document in 2011. Primary tenets of both documents include consumer control of data transfer to third parties, data security, and consent for collection of certain health and financial data. Neither framework, however, penalizes violators of the codes of conduct.

Privacy and Data Collection

Privacy regulation can require users' consent before an advertiser can track the user or communicate with the user. However, affirmative consent ("opt in") can be difficult and expensive to obtain. Industry participants often prefer other regulatory schemes.

Different jurisdictions have taken different approaches to privacy issues with advertising. The United States has specific restrictions on online tracking of children in the Children's Online Privacy Protection Act (COPPA), and the FTC has recently expanded its interpretation of COPPA to include requiring ad networks to obtain parental consent before knowingly tracking kids. Otherwise, the U.S. Federal Trade Commission frequently supports industry self-regulation, although increasingly it has been undertaking enforcement actions related to online privacy and security. The FTC has also been pushing for industry consensus about possible Do Not Track legislation.

In contrast, the European Union's "Privacy and Electronic Communications Directive" restricts websites' ability to use consumer data much more comprehensively. The EU limitations restrict targeting by online advertisers; researchers have estimated online advertising effectiveness decreases on average by around 65% in Europe relative to the rest of the world.

Delivery Methods

Many laws specifically regulate the ways online ads are delivered. For example, online advertising delivered via email is more regulated than the same ad content delivered via banner ads. Among other restrictions, the U.S. CAN-SPAM Act of 2003 requires that any commercial email provide an opt-out mechanism. Similarly, mobile advertising is governed by the Telephone Consumer Protection Act of 1991 (TCPA), which (among other restrictions) requires user opt-in before sending advertising via text messaging.

Integrated marketing Communication: (IMC)

Integrated marketing communication (IMC) is a conceptual approach used by the majority of organizations to develop a strategic plan on how they are going to broadcast their marketing and advertising campaigns. Recently there has been a shift in the way marketers and advertisers interact with their consumers and now see it as a conversation between Advertising/ Marketing teams and consumers. IMC has emerged as a key strategy for organizations to manage customer experiences in the digital age. The more traditional advertising practices such as newspapers, billboards, and magazines are still used but fail to have the same effect now as they did in previous years.

The importance of the IMC is to make the marketing process seamless for both the brand and the consumer. IMC attempts to meld all aspects of marketing into one cohesive piece. This includes sales promotion, advertising, public relations, direct marketing, and social media. The entire point of IMC is to have all of these aspects of marketing work together as a unified force. This can be done through methods, channels, and activities all while using a media platform. The end goal of IMC is to get the brands message across to consumers in the most convenient way possible.

Advantages of using IMC are that it has the ability to communicate the same message through several channels to create brand awareness. IMC is the most cost-effective solution when compared to mass media advertising to interact with target consumers on a personal level. IMC also benefits small businesses, as they are able to submerge their consumers with communication of various kinds in a way that pushes them through the research and buying stages creating a relationship and dialogue with their new customer. Popular and obvious examples of IMC put into action are the likes of direct marketing to the consumer that the organisation already has a knowledge that the person is interested in the brand by gathering personal information about them from when they previously shopped there and then sending mail, emails, texts and other direct communication with the person. In-store sales promotions are tactics such as '30% off' sales or offering loyalty cards to consumers to build a relationship. Television and radio advertisement are also a form of advertising strategy derived from IMC. All of the components of IMC play an important role and a company may or may not choose to implement any of the integration strategies

MEDIA CHANNELS

Media channels, also known as, marketing communications channels, are used to create a connection with the target consumer. Traditional methods of communication with the consumer include newspapers, magazines, Radio, television, billboards, telephone, post and door to door sales. These are just a few of the historically traditional methods.

Along with traditional media channels, comes new and upcoming media channels. Social media has begun to play a very large role in the way media and marketing intermingle to reach a consumer base. Social media has the power to reach a wider audience. Depending on the age group and demographic, social media can influence a company's overall image. Using social media as a marketing tool has become a widely popular method for branding. A brand has the chance to create an entire social media presence based around their own specific targeted community.

With advancements in digital communications channels, marketing communications allow for the possibility of two-way communications where an immediate consumer response can be elicited. Digital communications tools include: websites, blogs, social media, email, mobile, and search engines as a few examples. It is important for an advertising campaign to carefully select channels based on where their target consumer spends time to ensure market and advertising efforts are maximized.

Modern day implications to the advantages & disadvantages of traditional media channels

In the rapidly changing marketing and advertising environment, exposure to certain consumer groups and target audiences through traditional media channels has blurred. These traditional media channels are defined as print, broadcast, out-of-home and direct mail. The introduction of various new modern-day media channels has altered their traditional advantages and disadvantages. It is imperative to the effectiveness of the Integrated Marketing Communication (IMC) strategy that exposure to certain demographics, consumer groups and target audiences is anticipated to provide clarity, consistency, and maximum communications impact.

Print media is mainly defined as newspapers and magazines. With the transition in last decade [2006 – 2016] to digital information on phones, computers and tablets, the demographic that still are exposed to traditional print media is going to be older. It is also estimated that there will be a reduction of print material in coming years. This has to be taken into account by the advertisers and in some cases, they could use this to their advantage. Newspapers advantages would be that it is low cost, timely, reader controls exposure and has moderate coverage to the older generations in western society. Disadvantages would obviously be the aging demographic, short life, clutter and low attention-getting capabilities. Magazines are similar in some cases but have defined differences as they are a niche product increasing segmentation potential; they also have high informational content and longevity. Disadvantages are they are visual only, lack of flexibility and a long lead time for advertisement placement.

Traditional broadcast media's primary platforms are television and radio. These are still relatively prominent in modern-day society, but with the emergence of online content such as YouTube, Instagram and Vine it would difficult to anticipate where the market is headed in the next decade. Televisions advantages are that it has mass coverage, high reach, quality reputation, low post per exposure and impacts human senses. Disadvantages would be that it has low selectivity, short message life and high production costs. Alternatively, radio offers flexibility, high frequency and low advertising & production costs. Disadvantages to radio are that its audio only, low attention-getting and short message.

Out-of-home (OOH) media a broad marketing concept that is no longer relegated to large, static billboards on the side of motorways. More current and innovative approaches to OOH media range from street furniture to aerial blimps. Due to the constant and contemporary nature of the outdoors there will always be new ways in which a campaign can revitalize this media channel. Advantages would be the accessibility and reach, geographic flexibility and relatively low cost. Disadvantages to OOH media are that it has a short life, difficult to measure / control and it can convey poor brand image.

When an organisation begins to construct their advertising campaign they need to research each and every aspect of their target market and target consumer. The target consumer is the person or group of people who is most likely to buy from an organisation, he is also called 'potential customer'. A target consumer can be categorized by several key characteristics; Gender, age, occupation, marital status, geographical location, behavioral, level of income and education to name the main factors. This process is called segmenting customers on the basis of demographics.

Gender is simply whether a person is male or female. Age is usually broken up into bracketed intervals of ten or so years, for example, a person's age between 15–25 years old. By understanding which age bracket the target market falls into the advertisers can position their efforts accordingly. Occupation is also known as a profession and refers to what a person does for a living; this could be a particular job, student, unemployed etc. A person's marital status defines whether they are married or unmarried. Geographical location is a broad term specifying a particular area or place within a given country, state/ city, suburb or street as some examples. Income refers to how much money a person is earning annually which can help identify how much money they have left over after expenses to potential spend on a brand. The final factor to explain is education, whether a person went to school or not, what school they attended, what standard of education they have, diplomas, certificates, graduate, degrees, masters, Ph.D. or other forms of defining educational factors. Knowing this information can help an advertiser understand their target markets level of thinking to help adapt the advertising campaign to be understood by the given target consumer/s.

In advertising various brands compete to overtake the perceptual mapping in a consumers mind. Everyday consumers view advertising and rank particular brands compared to their competitors. Individuals rank these specific brands in an order of what is most important to them. For example, a person may compare brands of cars based on how sporty they think they look, affordability, practicality and classiness. How one person perceives a brand is different to another but is largely left to the advertising campaign to manipulate and create the perception that they want you to envision as the consumer.

Positioning is an important marketing concept that businesses implement to market their products or services. The positioning concept focuses on creating an image that will best attract the intended audience. Businesses that implement the positioning concept focus on promotion, price, placement and product. When the positioning concept is effective and productive it elevates the marketing efforts made by a business, and assists the buyer in purchasing the product.

The positioning process is imperative in marketing because of the specific level of consumer-based recognition is involved. A company must create a trademark brand for themselves in order to be recognizable by a broad range of consumers. For example, a fast food restaurant positions itself as fast, cheap, and delicious.

They are playing upon their strengths and most visible characteristics. On the other hand, a luxury car brand will position its brand as a stylish and expensive platform because they want to target a specific brand very different than the fast food brand.

For the positioning concept to be effective one must focus on the concepts of promotion, price, place and product.

There are three basic objectives of promotion, which include: presenting product information to targeted business customers and consumers, increase demand among the target market, and differentiating a product and creating a brand identity. Tools that can be used to achieve these objectives are advertising, public relations, personal selling, direct marketing, and sales promotion.

Price of an object is crucial in the concept of positioning. Adjusting or decreasing the product price has a profound impact on the sales of the product, and should complement the other parts of the positioning concept. The price needs to ensure survival, increase profit, generate survival, gain market shares, and establish an appropriate image.

Positioning a product is essential in the positioning concept. It is the process marketers use to communicate their products' attributes to the intended target market. In order for products to be successful businesses must focus on the customer needs, competitive pressures, available communication channels and carefully crafted key messages.

Product Positioning presents several advantages in the advertising campaign, and to the businesses/ individuals that implement it. Positioning connects with superior aspects of a product and matches "them with consumers more effectively than competitors" (Jaideep, S. 2016). Positioning can also help businesses or individuals realise the consumer's expectations of the product/s they are willing to purchase from them. Positioning a product reinforces the companies name, product and brand. It also makes the brand popular and strengthens customer loyalty. Product benefits to customers are better advertised through positioning the product, which results in more interest and attention of consumers. This also attracts different types of consumers as products posse's different benefits that attract different groups of consumers, for example: a shoe that is advertised for playing sports, going for walks, hiking and casual wear will attract different groups of consumers. Another advantage of positioning is the competitive strength it gives to businesses/ individuals and their products, introducing new products successfully to the market and communicating new and varied features that are added to a product later on.

Communication Process Diagram

The Communication of processes diagram refers to the order of operation an advertising campaign pieces together the flow of communication between a given organisation and the consumer. The diagram usually flows left to right (unless shown in a circular array) starting with the source. An advertising campaign uses the communication process diagram to ensure all the appropriate steps of communication are being taken in order.

The source is the person or organisation that has a message they want to share with potential consumers. An example of this is Vodafone wanting to tell their consumers and new consumers of a new monthly plan.

The diagram then moves on to encoding which consists of the organisation putting messages, thoughts and ideas into a symbolic form that be interpreted by the target consumer using symbols or words.

The third stage in the diagram is channel message. This occurs when the information or meaning the source wants to convoy, is put into a form to easily be transmitted to the targeted audience. This also includes the method that communication gets from the source to the receiver. Examples of this is Vodafone advertising on TV, bus stops and university campuses as students may be the intended consumer for the new plan.

Decoding is the processes that the viewer interprets the message that the source sent. Obviously it is up to the source to ensure that the message encoded well enough so that it is received as intended.

The receiver is also known as the viewer or potential consumer. This is the person who interprets the source message through channeling whether they are the intended target audience or not. Every day we interpret different advertisements even if we are not the target audience for that advertisement.

In between these steps there are external factors acting as distractions, these factors are called noise. Noise distorts the way the message gets to the intended target audience.These distractions are from all other forms of advertising and communication from every other person or organisation. Examples of noise are State of mind, unfamiliar language, unclear message, Values, Attitudes, Perceptions, Culture and Knowledge of similar products or services to name a few forms of noise.

Finally there is the response or feedback. This is the receiver's reaction to the communication of message and the way they understood it. Feedback relates to the way sales react as well as the interest or questions that arise in relation to the message put out.

Touch Points

When considering touch points in an advertising campaign a brand looks Multisensory touch points. These touch points help the brand to develop a point of contact between themselves and the consumer. Modern day advancements in various forms of technology have made it easier for consumers to engage with brands in numerous ways. The most successful touch points are those that create value in the consumer and brands relationship. Common examples of touch points include social media links, QR codes, person handing out flyers about a particular brand, billboards, web sites and various other methods that connect the brand and consumer.

Multi sensory touch points are subconscious yet helps use to recognise brands through characteristic identified through human sensors.These characteristics could be shape, colour, textures, sounds, smell or tastes associated with a given brand. It is important for an advertising campaign to consider sensory cues into their campaign as market places continue to become increasingly competitive and crowded. Anyone of the given sensory characteristics may remind a person of the brand they best associate with. A prime example of this is Red Bull who use the colour, shapes and size of their cans to best relate their product to success and winning. A taller can looks like the 1st place podium when placed next to competitors, the design looks like the finish flag in racing representing winning. The opportunity for an advertising campaign to succeed is significantly increased with the use of multi sensory touch points used as a point of difference between brands.

Guerrilla Marketing

Guerrilla marketing is an advertising strategy which increases brand exposure through the use of unconventional campaigns which initiate social discussion and "buzz". This can often be achieved with lower budgets than conventional advertising methods, allowing small and medium-sized businesses the chance to compete against larger competitors. Through unconventional methods, inventiveness and creativity, guerrilla marketing leaves the receiver with a long lasting impression of the brand as most guerrilla marketing campaigns target the receivers at a personal level, taking them by surprise and may incorporate an element of shock. Guerrilla marketing is typically executed exclusively in public places, including streets, parks, shopping centres etc., to ensure maximum audience resulting in further discussion on social media.

Guerrilla marketing is the term used for several types of marketing categories including street marketing, ambient marketing, presence marketing, alternative marketing, experimental marketing, grassroots marketing, wild posting, guerrilla projection advertising, undercover marketing and astroturfing.

Jay Conrad Levinson coined the term Guerrilla Marketing with his 1984 book of the same name. Through the enhancement of technology and common use of internet and mobile phones, marketing communication has become more affordable and guerrilla marketing is on the rise, allowing the spread of newsworthy guerrilla campaigns.

When establishing a guerrilla marketing strategy, there are seven elements to a clear and logical approach. Firstly, write a statement that identifies the purpose of the strategy. Secondly define how the purpose will be achieved concentrating on the key advantages. Next Levinson (1989) suggests writing a descriptive summary on the target market or consumers. The fourth element is to establish a statement that itemizes the marketing tools and methods planning to be used in the strategy (for example, radio advertising during 6.30am – 9am on weekday mornings or window displays that are regularly updated). The fifth step is to create a statement which positions the brand/product/company in the market. Define the brands characteristics and give it an identity is the sixth element. Lastly, clearly identify a budget which will be put solely towards marketing going forward.

For a successful overall guerrilla marketing campaign, combine the above steps with seven winning actions. These seven principles are commitment – stick to the marketing plan without changing it; investment – appreciate that marketing is an investment, consistency – ensure the marketing message and strategy remains consistent across all forms of, confidence – show confidence in the commitment to the guerrilla marketing strategy, patience – time and dedication to the strategy, assortment – incorporate different methods of advertising and marketing for optimum results, and subsequent – build customer loyalty and retention though follow up marketing post-sale.

Levinson suggests guerrilla marketing tactics were initiated to enable small businesses with limited financial resources to gain an upper hand on the corporate giants who had unlimited budgets and resources at their disposal. Large companies cottoned on to the success of guerrilla marketing and have had hundreds of effective attention grabbing campaigns using the strategies originally designed for smaller businesses with minimal marketing budgets.

Non-traditional, unconventional and shocking campaigns are highly successful in obtaining media coverage and therefore brand awareness, albeit good or bad media attention. However, like most marketing strategies a bad campaign can backfire and damage profits and sales. Undercover marketing and astroturfing are two type of guerrilla marketing that are deemed as risky and can be detrimental to the company.

"Advertising can be dated back to 4000 BC where Egyptians used papyrus to make sales messages and wall posters. Traditional advertising and marketing slowly developed over the centuries but never bloomed until early 1900s" ("What Is Guerrilla Marketing?", 2010). Guerrilla marketing are relatively simple, use tactics to advertise on a very small budget. It is to make a campaign that is "shocking, funny, unique, outrageous, clever and creative that people can't stop talking about it" (Uk essays, 2016). Guerrilla marketing is different when compared to traditional marketing tactics (Staff, 2016). "Guerrilla marketing means going after conventional goals of profits, sales and growth but doing it by using unconventional means, such as expanding offerings during gloomy economic days to inspire customers to increase the size of each purchase" (Staff, 2016). Guerrilla marketing also suggests that rather than investing money, it is better to "invest time, energy, imagination and knowledge" (Staff, 2016) instead. Guerrilla marketing puts profit as their main priority not sales as their main focal point, this is done to urge the growth of geometrically by enlarging the size of each transactions. This all done through one of the most powerful marketing weapons around, the telephone. Research shows that it will always increases profits and sales. The term "guerrilla first appeared during the war of independence in Spain and Portugal at the beginning of the 19th century it can be translated as battle" (Uk essays, 2016). Even thou guerrilla marketing was aimed for small business; this did not stop bigger business from adopting the same ideology. "Larger business has been using unconventional marketing to complement their advertising campaigns, even then some marketers argue that when bigger business utilize guerrilla marketing tactics, it isn't true guerrilla" ("What Is Guerrilla Marketing?", 2010).

The reason being that larger companies have bigger budgets and usually their brands well established. In some cases, it is far riskier for a larger business to do guerrilla marketing tactics. Which can cause problem when their stunts become a flop when compared to smaller business, as they do not run as much risk, as most people will just write it off as another failed stunt. Many methods in guerrilla marketing consist of "graffiti (or reverse graffiti, where a dirty wall is selectively cleaned), interactive displays, intercept encounters in public spaces, flash mobs, or various PR stunts are often used."

Small business use social media as a form of marketing. This Is due to that social media in the 21st century is phenomenon. "Collecting billions of people around the world through a series of status updates, tweets, and other rich media" ("Guerrilla Marketing Strategies for Small Businesses", 2013). Social media is a powerful tool in the world of business. Guerrilla marketing strategies and tactics are a great and cost effective way to generate" awareness for your business, products and services. To maximize full potential in your marketing efforts, it's to blend them with a powerful and robust online marking strategy with a marketing automation software" ("Guerrilla Marketing Strategies for Small Businesses", 2013). Which can boost small businesses. Guerrilla tactics consist of instruments that have effects on the efforts. Some instruments are usually there to maximize the surprise effect and some of these instruments mainly cutting advertising costs." Guerrilla marketing is a way of increasing the number of individuals exposed to the advertising with the cost of campaign. The instrument of diffusion helps to each a wide audience, which causes none or little cost because consumers (viral marketing) or the media (guerrilla PR) pass on the advertising message" ("Guerrilla Marketing:

The Nature of the Concept and Propositions for Further Research", 2016). Guerrilla campaigns usually implement a free ride approach, this means that to cut their costs and increase the number of recipients simultaneously to maximize the low cost effect. For example, they will try to benefit from placing advertisements on big events e.g. sporting events. Guerrilla marketing was regarded to target existing customers rather than new ones, aiming to increase their engagement with a product and/ or brand. "When selecting audiences for a guerrilla message, a group that is already engaged with the product at some level is the best target; they will be quicker to recognize and respond to creative tactics, and more likely to share the experience with their friends, as social media has become a major feature of the market landscape, guerrilla marketing has shown to be particularly effective online. Consumers who regularly use social media are more likely to share their interactions with guerrilla marketing, and creative advertising can quickly go viral."

Direct-To-Consumer Advertising

Direct-to-consumer advertising (DTCA) refers to the marketing and advertising of pharmaceutical products directly to consumers as patients, as opposed to specifically targeting health professionals. The term is synonymous primarily with the advertising of prescription medicines via mass media platforms—most commonly on television and in magazines, but also via online platforms.

Direct-to-consumer advertising is only completely legal in New Zealand and the United States, but are subject to regulations regarding the balanced disclosure of a prescription's benefits in comparison to its risks (including but not limited to side effects and contraindications), among other factors. Regulations regarding DTCA are typically applied to advertising materials that describe a prescription's indications and benefits, and may be more lenient to advertising materials which do not discuss uses. Many countries ban any advertising of prescription drugs directly to consumers.

There are ethical and regulatory concerns regarding DTCA, specifically the extent to which these ads may unduly influence the prescribing of the prescriptions based on consumer demands when, in some cases, they may not be medically necessary, or there are cheaper options available. Critics of DTCA have argued that too much is spent on marketing medications, rather than into research and development; in the United States, ad spending by drugmakers reached US$5.2 billion in 2016.

Types

The U.S. Food and Drug Administration (FDA) defines several common types of DTCA for prescription medication:

A "product claim" advertisement identifies the nonproprietary and trade names of the medication, and contains at least one approved indication, and claims surrounding its benefits.

A "reminder" advertisement is designed to build brand recognition for a medication. Reminder ads cannot contain any information or imagery that pertain to the medication's approved uses, but may have themes that vaguely allude to them; for example, a reminder commercial for the erectile dysfunction drug Viagra featured the showtune "Good Morning" and scenes of a man happily walking to work, emphasizing a sexual innuendo in the lyric "it's great to stay up late". They may still contain a call to action urging viewers to ask their doctor or seek an external resource (such as a website or phone hotline) for more information.

A "help-seeking" advertisement is not presented as marketing for a drug first and foremost, and instead resemble an awareness campaign for a specific medical condition. They do not specify any specific product or treatment, and direct the audience to ask their doctor or seek an external resource for more information. These outlets are, in turn, used to promote specific prescription options. Help-seeking campaigns are sometimes used as preliminary marketing for new drugs.

Reminder and help-seeking ads are often used by drugmakers to bypass the more onerous restrictions (such as the required listing of side effects), or outright prohibitions on product claims advertising, as neither of them are focused on promoting the drug itself. Sometimes, a campaign may mix both of these ads, with one ad discussing the condition, and another, similarly-styled ad, mentioning the product but not the condition, seeking to have the viewer infer the association between the ads.

Legality

Brazil

In 2008 a new resolution from ANVISA (Control Agency for Sanitary Vigilance), Resolution 96 from December 17 was released, with focus on medication advertisements. It allows direct-to-consumer advertising of non-prescription medication, with restrictions on the type of drug and words and images that can be used, among other things. Advertisements for prescription medications can only appear in scientific, medical, or health professional journals.

Canada

The Food and Drugs Act prohibits most direct-to-consumer advertising of prescription medications: all direct-to-consumer advertising of drugs was forbidden until 1978, when Health Canada began to allow ads containing names, quantities, and prices only, so that pharmacies could display their prices for comparison purposes. In 2000, Health Canada adopted an interpretation of this law allowing for the aforementioned "reminder" and "help-seeking" advertisements, although U.S.-style "full product ads" that mention the purpose of a prescription remain prohibited. Later that year, Health Canada ruled that a pairing of similarly-themed reminder and help-seeking commercials ran afoul of the regulations, as their combination constituted a full product ad.

There are no regulations requiring direct-to-consumer marketing prohibited under Canadian law to be removed or substituted from U.S. television channels and print publications distributed in the country.

In 2014, York University professor and physician Dr. Joel Lexchin, and University of British Columbia associate professor Barbara Mintzes, published a study that highlighted 10 DTC cases between 2000 and 2011 with "unsatisfactory" responses from Health Canada. They found that Health Canada's application of these regulations "[lacked] accountability and transparency"—with no public record of complaints and enforcement besides media coverage of certain prominent cases, and no evidence that Health Canada has ever issued fines for violations. In conclusion, they stated that "since DTCA became prominent in the U.S. in the mid-1990s, successive governments of different political stripes in Canada have shown a remarkably consistent commitment to non-enforcement".

Europe

In October 2002, the European Commission voted against a proposal to selectively allow advertising of "disease education information" in relation to AIDS, asthma, and diabetes. Despite insistence otherwise due to its selective and controlled nature, the European Parliament Committee on the Environment, Public Health and Food Safety assessed that the pharmaceutical industry could not be trusted to provide impartial and unbiased information. UK Labour Party MEP Catherine Stihler argued that the proposal was a "slippery slope" towards U.S.-style advertising practices promoting expensive "wonder drugs", and that "we don't want consumers sitting on their couches bombarded with a hard sell from big drug companies in the advertising break between Crossroads and Coronation Street."

Bibliography

- Medicare Expenditures for Pimavanserin. Psychiatric Services. 72 (1): 77–80. doi:10.1176/appi.ps.202000251. PMID 32838675. S2CID 221308577.
- Glossary Term: Key Opinion Leader. Pharma Marketing Network.
- Finding Key Opinion Leaders Using Social Network Analysis (PDF). Lnx Research. 2007. Archived from the original (PDF) on 12 July 2011.
- Myers KD. Marketing to Professionals: Tomorrow's Changes Today. www.pharmexec.com. Archived from the original on 17 December 2007.
- GlaxoSmithKline to Plead Guilty and Pay $3 Billion to Resolve Fraud Allegations and Failure to Report Safety Data. 2 July 2012. Archived from the original on 9 September 2014. Retrieved 22 November 2020.
- JUSTICE DEPARTMENT ANNOUNCES LARGEST HEALTH CARE FRAUD (PDF). US department of Justice. Archived (PDF) from the original on 2 December 2020. Retrieved 19 May 2016.
- Abbott Labs to Pay $1.5 Billion to Resolve Criminal & Civil Investigations of Off-label Promotion of Depakote. 7 May 2012. Archived from the original on 21 August 2014. Retrieved 22 November 2020.
- #09-038: Eli Lilly and Company Agrees to Pay $1.415 Billion to Resolve Allegationsof Off-label Promotion of Zyprexa (2009-01-15). Archived from the original on 13 March 2016. Retrieved 22 November 2020.
- Drazen, Jeffrey M. (2015). Revisiting the Commercial–Academic Interface. New England Journal of Medicine. 372 (19): 1853–1854. doi:10.1056/NEJMe1503623. PMID 25946285.
- Rosenbaum, Lisa (2015). Reconnecting the Dots — Reinterpreting Industry–Physician Relations. New England Journal of Medicine. 372 (19): 1860–1864. doi:10.1056/NEJMms1502493. PMID 25946288.

- Covid vaccine front-runners: How much they cost, who's bought them and how they're stored. CNBC. 17 November 2020. Archived from the original on 1 December 2020. Retrieved 2 December 2020.
- No profiteering on COVID-19 drugs and vaccines, says MSF. Médecins Sans Frontières (MSF) International. Archived from the original on 26 November 2021. Retrieved 22 April 2020.
- HHS, DOD Collaborate with Regeneron on Large-Scale Manufacturing Demonstration Project of COVID-19 Investigational Therapeutic Treatment. 6 July 2020. Archived from the original on 18 December 2020. Retrieved 2 December 2020.
- Gardner AW, Afaq A (2008). Management of Lower Extremity Peripheral Arterial Disease. Journal of Cardiopulmonary Rehabilitation and Prevention. 28 (6): 349–57. doi:10.1097/HCR.0b013e31818c3b96. PMC 2743684. PMID 19008688.
- Craig WM (1939). Surgical Treatment of Hypertension. Br Med J. 2 (4120): 1215–9. doi:10.1136/bmj.2.4120.1215. PMC 2178707. PMID 20782854.
- Sneader, Walter (2005). Drug Discovery. A History. New York: Wiley. p. 371.
- Beyer KH (1993). Chlorothiazide. How the thiazides evolved as antihypertensive therapy. Hypertension. 22 (3): 388–91. doi:10.1161/01.hyp.22.3.388. PMID 8349332.
- BORHANI NO, HECHTER HH (1964). Recent Changes in CVR Disease Mortality in California: An Epidemiologic Appraisal. Public Health Rep. 79 (2): 147–60. doi:10.2307/4592077. JSTOR 4592077. PMC 1915335. PMID 14119789.
- The Lasker Foundation - Awards. Archived from the original on 23 December 2015. Retrieved 24 February 2022.
- Black JW, Crowther AF, Shanks RG, Smith LH, Dornhorst AC (1964). A new adrenergic betareceptor antagonist. The Lancet. 283 (7342): 1080–1081. doi:10.1016/S0140-6736(64)91275-9. PMID 14132613.
- Lv J, Perkovic V, Foote CV, Craig ME, Craig JC, Strippoli GF (2012). Antihypertensive agents for preventing diabetic kidney disease. Cochrane Database Syst Rev. 12: CD004136. doi:10.1002/14651858.CD004136.pub3. PMID 23235603.
- A brief history of the birth control pill - The pill timeline | Need to Know | PBS. PBS. 7 May 2010. Archived from the original on 19 January 2018. Retrieved 8 September 2017.

INDEX

T

V

9 788197 595738

Printed at Repro India Ltd.